NUTRITARIAN HANDBOOK
& ANDI* FOOD SCORING GUIDE

ANDI = Aggregate Nutrient Density Index

OTHER BOOKS BY
Joel Fuhrman, M.D.

End of Diabetes–
The Eat to Live Plan to Prevent and Reverse Diabetes

The Eat to Live Cookbook–
Over 180 Nutrient-Rich Recipes
Plus Cooking and Food Purchasing Tips

Eat For Health–
Lose Weight • Keep it Off • Look Younger • Live Longer

The New York Times Best Seller
Super Immunity–
The Essential Guide for Boosting Your Body's Defenses
to Live Longer, Stronger, and Disease Free

The New York Times #1 Best Seller
Eat to Live–
The Revolutionary Formula for
Fast and Sustained Weight Loss

Disease-Proof Your Child–
Feeding Kids Right

Fasting and Eating for Health–
A Medical Doctor's Program for Conquering Disease

www.DrFuhrman.com
Dr. Fuhrman's official website for information,
recipes, supportive services, and products

Nutritarian Handbook
AND ANDI FOOD SCORING GUIDE

JOEL FUHRMAN, M.D.

PUBLISHED BY

qþ

Gift of Health Press

Contact:
Gift of Health Press
Flemington, NJ 08822
for wholesale inquiries go to:
giftofhealthpress.com

Printed in the United States of America
ISBN-13: 978-0-9837952-1-6
Library of Congress Control Number: 2011941079

Publisher's Note:
Do not start, stop, or change medication without professional
medical advice, and do not change your diet if you are ill or on
medication, except under the supervision of a competent physician.
Neither this, nor any other book, is intended to take the place of
personalized medical care or treatment.

ထ

Gift of Health Press

Book Design — Robyn Rolfes, Creative Syndicate, Inc.

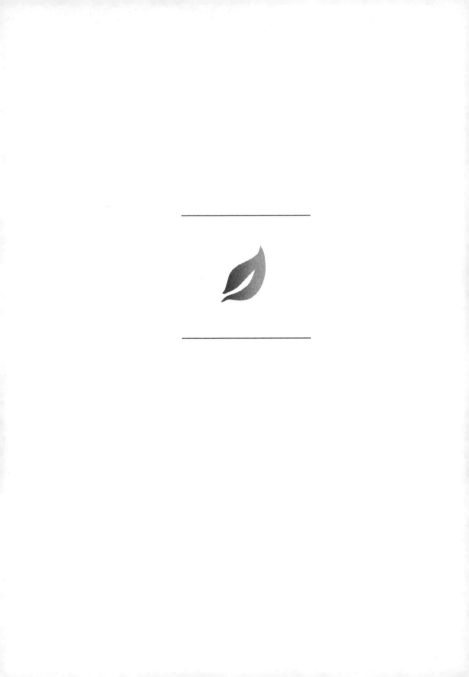

CONTENTS

INTRODUCTION

No one wants to have a heart attack, suffer a debilitating stroke or develop cancer. But lots of people die from these conditions every day... unnecessarily.

Nutritional science has made dramatic advances in recent years. The overwhelming accumulation of scientific knowledge points to a dramatic conclusion—the majority of diseases plaguing Americans are preventable. Using the information compiled from scientific studies, it is now possible to formulate a few simple diet and lifestyle principles that can save you years of suffering and premature death. You have an unprecedented opportunity in human history to enjoy better health and live longer than ever before.

But being in the best of health and living longer comes at a price.

How much would it be worth to you for a guarantee that you would never have a heart attack or a stroke? What would it be worth to you to healthfully and happily watch your children and grandchildren grow? What would you be willing to pay for the assurance that you would not leave your spouse or your children all alone?

Fortunately, the expenditure is infinitely affordable—little more than the effort needed to establish new, more healthful eating habits.

Everything in this book is supported by the preponderance of evidence from scientific studies. Still, the facts and guidelines will astound most physicians. Although the research is readily available for all to see, most people still have no idea that food can be the most powerful weapon in the fight against the major illnesses that plague our society. Now is the time for you to open your eyes to the value of superior nutrition, put wholesome food in your body and take control of your health destiny.

CHAPTER ONE

AMERICA'S HEALTH CRISIS AND YOU

Americans are digging their graves with their knives and forks. It is not news that Americans are sickly and fat. Almost everybody knows modern America is in the midst of an all-you-can eat food fest that has us literally busting at the seams. We are not only eating ourselves into sickness and premature death, but we also have a health care crisis with upward spiraling medical care costs.

The economic costs of heart disease and other diet-related chronic diseases are staggering. Health care costs increased over 50 percent between 2000 and 2005 and now our nation's medical costs exceed 2.4 trillion, over 4 times the amount spent on national defense. The annual healthcare cost of obesity in the US has doubled in less than a decade and may be as high as 147 billion dollars a year. The medical costs for an obese person are 42% higher than for a person of normal weight.[1] These out-of-control costs play an important role in business failures, bankruptcies and loss of jobs.

Our health system relies on an ever-expanding arsenal of medications, tests and procedures that fail to address the *root cause* of our escalating ill health—the way we choose to eat and live. In America, we have attempted to solve our dietary-caused health woes with the development of multiple medications for diabetes, hypertension and cholesterol-lowering. We have tried heart procedures and surgeries, all at a dramatic expense. We have been led to believe that drugs and doctors save lives, but the statistics show otherwise; lifespan is not significantly enhanced by the vast majority of medical interventions.

The Obesity Epidemic

Nutritionally-caused disease is now the largest cause of death throughout the world and for the first time globally, the number of overweight individuals rivals the number of those who are underweight. In recent years, the growth of processed foods, convenience foods and fast foods has supplied our relatively sedentary society with a diet of high calorie foods with few nutrients.

In all parts of the world, obesity appears to escalate as income increases and fast food and processed foods become available. Nowhere has this problem become as large as in America where we have the biggest waistlines in the world. In the United States, being overweight is the norm and almost all adults eventually take medications for their heart, diabetes, cholesterol or blood pressure.

The number of obese Americans is higher than the number of those who smoke, use illegal drugs or suffer from other physical ailments. Obesity is a major risk factor associated with highly prevalent and serious diseases, such as heart disease, cancer and diabetes. The diet-style that creates these diseases fuels out-of-control medical costs.

The average woman in America today weighs 40 pounds more than women did 100 years ago and has a considerably higher risk of heart attack, stroke and breast cancer to show for it. The rate of sudden cardiac death for the average American male has quadrupled in the past 100 years, and his risk of heart attack is ten times higher. Both sexes, on average, are 30 pounds heavier today than they were in the 1960's. But it is not all about weight. It is much worse than that.

Health Complications of Obesity

- Increased overall mortality
- Adult onset diabetes
- Hypertension
- Degenerative arthritis
- Coronary artery disease
- Obstructive sleep apnea
- Gallstones
- Fatty infiltration of liver
- Restrictive lung disease
- Cancer

Poor Nutrition Everywhere

In the 20th century, processed foods became increasingly prevalent in the average American diet. The consumption of fresh produce and whole grains plummeted while the consumption of animal products increased. As a result, Americans now consume far more calories, fat, cholesterol, refined sugar, animal protein, sodium, white flour and far less fiber and plant-derived nutrients than is healthful. Obesity, diabetes, heart disease and cancer have skyrocketed.

CHANGE IN FOOD CONSUMPTION IN THE LAST 100 YEARS IN THE UNITED STATES

	1900	2000
Sugar	5 lbs/year	170 lbs/year
Soft drinks	0	53 gallons/year
Oils	4 lbs/year	74 lbs/year
Cheese	2 lbs/year	30 lbs/year
Meat	140 lbs/year	200 lbs/year
Homegrown Produce	131 lbs/year	11 pounds/year
Calories	2100	2757

Our society has evolved to a level of economic sophistication that allows us to eat ourselves to death. A diet centered on milk, cheese, pasta, bread, fried foods, sugar-filled snacks and drinks lays the groundwork for obesity, cancer, heart disease, diabetes and autoimmune illnesses. It is not solely that these foods are harmful; it is also what we are not eating that is causing the problem. We are not eating enough nutrient-rich produce.

When you calculate all the calories consumed from the Standard American Diet, you find that the calories coming from the most health-promoting foods, such as fresh fruit, vegetables, beans, raw nuts, and seeds, are less than ten percent of the total caloric intake. This dangerously low intake of unrefined plant foods is what guarantees weakened immunity to infectious disease, frequent illnesses and a shorter lifespan. We will never win the war on cancer, heart disease, diabetes, and other degenerative illnesses unless we address this deficiency. Though the American diet has spread all over the world, bringing with it heart disease, cancer and obesity, studies still show that in the populations that eat more fruits and vegetables, the incidences of death from these diseases is dramatically lowered.[2]

COMPOSITION OF THE AMERICAN DIET

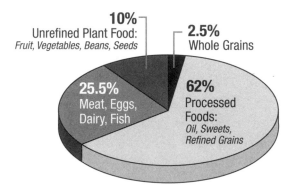

United States Department of Agriculture Economics Research Service, 2005.
http://www.ers.usda.gov/Data/FoodConsuption/FoodGuideIndex.htm#calories

Heart Disease is Preventable

Heart disease is a much bigger problem than most people think. Heart attacks and strokes are the cause of death for almost one-third of all Americans. Yet, heart disease is a relatively new phenomenon in human history and is easy to prevent.

One hundred years ago, heart disease affected less than 5 percent of the population. Today, it affects almost all Americans, with more than 45 percent of our population over the age of 65 taking cholesterol lowering drugs.[3] It is estimated that 90 percent of Americans age 65 and over take some sort of prescription drugs daily.[4] Modern medical techniques and drugs cannot win this war because the true cause of disease is overlooked. Heart disease and most other common modern diseases are caused by inadequate nutrition.

The tragedy is enormous. More than 1.4 million Americans will suffer a heart attack this year.[5] When you consider that nobody really has to die from a heart- or circulatory-system-related death, it is even more of a tragedy. The disability, suffering and years of life lost are almost totally the result of dietary ignorance. It is not impossible or even difficult to protect yourself; you simply must eat properly. Nothing else can offer such dramatic protection.

DEATHS FROM DISEASES OF THE HEART

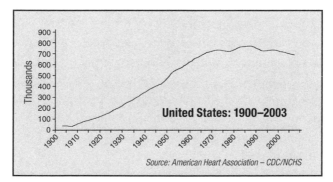

United States: 1900–2003

Source: American Heart Association – CDC/NCHS

4 Simple Truths

While America's health crisis is real, you can reclaim your health. Consider these four critical points:

- We are brainwashed into thinking that drugs are the answer to our health problems

- Unhealthy food is addictive

- Foods that don't contain health-promoting micronutrients lead to overeating

- A normal body weight in conjunction with nutritional adequacy is essential for good health and longevity

Understanding these simple truths is the key to solving the health care problems of most Americans.

The fact is, our bodies' cells need a wide array of nutrients numbering in the thousands to function normally. The human body is designed to be fueled by natural, nutrient-rich plant food. Foods supply not just vitamins and minerals, but thousands of immune-supporting substances called phytochemicals that are essential for our protection against disease.

While science has described these needs, an astonishing 95 percent of Americans do not even meet the Center for Disease Control's (CDC's) minimum nutritional guidelines for all the basic vitamins and minerals.[6] Very few people eat healthfully enough to protect themselves against disease in later life.

Why Diets Fail
Low-nutrient eating drives overeating behavior and is the primary cause of obesity, disease and death in the modern world.

Have you ever been on a diet, losing and gaining the same 10, 20 or 30 pounds? Research shows that over 95 percent of all weight lost on a "fad diet" is regained. The biggest problem with most diets is that you are asked to deprive yourself – portion control, low carbs, fewer calories, etc. Deprivation never works and your food cravings return with a vengeance! This unfortunately is the basis of the 'yo-yo' dieting industry. I want you to know that it's not that you have failed a diet; it's that the system (diets, magic pills, surgeries, etc.) has failed you.

My findings, based on my 20 years of experience with over 10,000 patients and thousands of supportive research studies are that a properly nourished body will seek its ideal weight. So instead of 'dieting', I want to show you the foods that provide the nutrition your body needs. **The body has an incredible ability to heal itself and get back in balance when you feed it what it needs. It's that simple!** Your body is like a supercomputer; feed it right and it will keep you fit, lean and healthy.

Enjoy a Full, More Pleasurable Life

If you are reading this, it is likely that you are someone who is ready to take control of your health. Superior Nutrition is the foundation of this diet. It is the path to medical wellness in your life. It is the most powerful intervention, not only to prevent disease, but to also reverse it. Complete recovery from most chronic degenerative illnesses is possible.

The information presented here is the fastest and most effective way to create an optimal nutritional environment for self-healing. This plant-based, high-nutrient dense diet can enable you to avoid angioplasty, bypass surgery and other invasive procedures. By adopting this eating style, you can make sure that you never have a heart attack, stroke or dementia. You can reduce and eventually eliminate your need for prescription drugs. You will not only optimize your health and potentially save your life, but this eating style will also increase the pleasure you get from food.

It will result in the lessening of hunger, the removal of addiction and if needed, profound and long-term weight loss. I have seen this in my medical practice and it has been documented in medical publications.[7] You will not only reach your ideal body weight, but you will enjoy a longer, more healthful and pleasurable life. More and more, new medical studies are investigating and demonstrating that diets rich in high-nutrient plant foods have a suppressive effect on appetite and are most effective for long-term weight control.[8] The healthiest way to eat is also the most successful way to obtain a favorable weight, if you consider long term results

I am thrilled to be able to work with you and address your diet-related health issues. You will learn how to feed your body so it operates at its highest level every day. Your energy levels will be amazing, without relying on artificial stimulants like coffee and sugar. You will sleep better, your skin will look better and you will feel and look younger. In short, your properly nourished body will allow you to live life to the fullest!

I encourage you to read my books, *Eat to Live* or *Eat for Health* for a more comprehensive understanding and application of these principles. I also offer an assortment of valuable membership features at DrFuhrman.com where you can obtain more detailed and personalized health and nutritional guidance.

BECOMING A NUTRITARIAN

Not Your Typical Diet

Typical diet books usually contain a list of rules and regulations to restrict calories for weight loss. This is a problem, because when the focus is weight loss alone, results are rarely permanent.

The focus in this handbook is on nutrition and *eating healthfully*, which is an undisputed, yet often overlooked critical ingredient to any dietary success. Here, there is no carbohydrate, protein or calorie counting, portion-size measuring or weighing involved. In fact, you will eat as much food as you want, and still over time you will become healthier and will be satisfied with fewer calories. A properly nourished body will *automatically seek its ideal weight*, without having to fight the scale or count calories.

The fundamentals of this eating style are to increase high-nutrient foods in your diet and to 'crowd out' unhealthful low-nutrient foods. What does it mean to crowd-out? It means that as you eat more delicious, high-nutrient foods, you will be reducing your desire for fatty, processed and unhealthful products.

When you change the foods you eat to better meet your nutrient needs, you feel better and it eventually becomes your preferred way of eating. To accomplish this, you will be presented with scientific, logical information that explains the connection between food and your weight and health. If you need to lose weight, this information will help you shed pounds naturally and easily, merely as a side effect of eating so healthfully.

What is a Nutritarian?
When you learn and practice this eating style, you can proudly call yourself a Nutritarian. A Nutritarian is someone who strives to consume and learns to prefer foods that are nutritious. Quite simply, a Nutritarian:

- Eats mainly high-nutrient, natural plant foods: vegetables, fruits, beans, nuts and seeds.

- Eats few, if any, animal products (one or two servings per week at most) and chooses healthier options in this food group.

- Eats almost no foods that are completely empty of nutrients or toxic for the body such as: sugar, sweeteners, white flour, processed foods and fast foods.

The Nutritarian way to health, longevity and weight loss focuses on healthy foods such as green vegetables, other colorful vegetables, fruits, beans, nuts and seeds.

A Nutritarian is someone who learns to trust the amazing power of the body. *If given half a chance, the body will heal itself*—with the right food as the catalyst. When you learn how to become a Nutritarian, you will arm yourself with the biochemical sustenance that your body needs to be at its ideal weight and to live a healthy, empowered life.

Finally, a Nutritarian lifestyle is an attitude, a mindset, a method that can be followed for a lifetime. As you begin your journey as a Nutritarian, you will be empowered to take control of your own health and life.

Vegetarian, Flexitarian or Nutritarian
The foundation of the Nutritarian diet is vegetables and other high-nutrient foods, but it does not have to be at the exclusion of all animal foods. A vegan diet is one that contains no foods of animal product origin whereas a vegetarian diet may contain some dairy and eggs. A vegetarian/vegan diet can be an option for excellent health as long as care is taken to eat healthful, nutrient-rich foods. However, a vegetarian/vegan who lives on processed cereals, white flour products, white rice, white potato and processed soy products is still vulnerable to the weight gain, diseases and many of the other complications resulting from the standard American diet because their diet cannot be considered nutrient-rich.

Being a Nutritarian differs from being a typical vegetarian because the focus isn't on totally excluding animal foods. The focus is on including the high-nutrient foods a body needs to improve health dramatically. A Nutritarian can reduce the level of animal products to a safe level without having to exclude them completely. A Nutritarian could be a vegan or not. Eating this way makes either option healthful.

The Nutritarian Difference
The Nutritarian diet is different because it doesn't require deprivation, starvation or denying your body foods that properly nourish it. It truly is a whole new way of looking at food. This handbook will show you why nutrient-rich foods are so powerful and will help you learn exactly what to eat and how to incorporate these foods into your diet.

Your body can change in amazing and dramatic ways. Many people who have adopted the Nutritarian lifestyle have reversed diet-related diseases such as diabetes, heart disease, chronic fatigue, autoimmune disease and migraines. The right food can be the most healing 'medicine' you put in your body.

I have developed a Nutritarian Food Plate© which illustrates what your plate should look like. It is comprised of the nutrient-rich plant foods according to their nutrient composition and disease-protective properties. These foods include raw and cooked vegetables, fruit, beans, nuts, seeds and whole grains. They should fill up most of your plate.

Poultry, eggs, dairy, fish, oil and white potato should comprise ten percent or less of your diet. Cheese, sweets, red meat, processed foods, white rice and flour should be eaten rarely, if at all. These foods provide few antioxidants and phytochemicals and decrease the nutrient density of your diet. Significant quantities of "high protein" foods also drive up hormones linked to higher rates of breast, prostate and colon cancer.

Dr. Fuhrman's Nutritarian Food Plate©

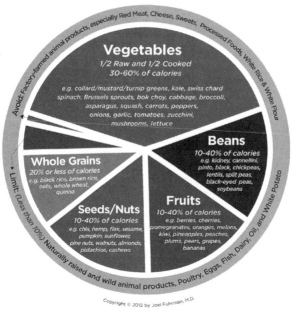

Copyright © 2012 by Joel Fuhrman, M.D.

CHAPTER THREE

THE HEALTH EQUATION

Discovering Nutrients

There are two kinds of nutrients: macronutrients and micronutrients. Macronutrients are protein, carbohydrate, fat (and water). Excluding water, they basically are the three calorie-containing nutrients.

Micronutrients are vitamins, minerals and phytochemicals and are calorie-free. Obviously, we need to consume both kinds of nutrients, but the American diet contains too many macronutrients and not enough micronutrients.

MACRONUTRIENTS = FAT, CARBOHYDRATE & PROTEIN
CONTAIN CALORIES
SHOULD LIMIT CONSUMPTION

MICRONUTRIENTS = VITAMINS, MINERALS & PHYTOCHEMICALS
DO NOT CONTAIN CALORIES
SHOULD INCREASE CONSUMPTION

Eating foods that are naturally rich in micronutrients is the secret to achieving optimal health and super immunity. A micronutrient-heavy diet supplies your body with 14 different vitamins, 25 different minerals, and more than 10,000 phytochemicals, which are plant-based chemicals that have profound effects on human cell function and the immune system. Foods that are naturally rich in these nutrients are also rich in fiber and water and are naturally low in calories, meaning they have a low caloric density. These low-calorie, high-nutrient foods provide the ingredients that activate your body's self-healing and self-repairing mechanisms. They are nature's contribution to your health turnaround! The foundational principle of this program is that the right food is your best medicine.

About 80 years ago, when scientists first identified vitamins and minerals, they thought they could have a profound effect on reducing risks of cancer and other life-shortening diseases. When the fortification of foods and the explosion of the supplement industry became a major contributor to America's micronutrient pie, an amazing thing happened. Cancer rates increased for 70 years straight from 1935 to 2005.[9] Cancer incidence and mortality rates are continuing to climb worldwide. Certainly, I am not suggesting the ingestion of these micronutrients was primarily to blame, but I am saying that vitamins and minerals alone are definitely not the answer.

We found out about 15 years ago that the major micronutrient load in food was NOT vitamins and minerals; it was phytochemicals. Shockingly, natural foods contained many more critical nutritional elements than was ever imagined. With thousands of nutrients in a strawberry or piece of broccoli, nutrient intake is more intricate then originally thought. When the right assortment of natural foods is consumed, these nutrients work harmoniously to increase our immunity and protect our body against disease.

The phytochemical revolution

All the different types of nutrients are vital to achieving and maintaining optimal health and nutritional excellence; however, phytochemicals hold a special, elite place in the nutritional landscape. When consistently consumed in adequate quantity and variety, phytochemicals become super-nutrients in your body. They work together to detoxify cancer-causing compounds, deactivate free radicals, protect against radiation damage and enable DNA repair mechanisms.[10] When altered or broken strands of DNA are repaired, it can prevent cancer from developing later in life.

Consuming phytochemicals is not optional. They are essential in human immune-system defenses. Without a wide variety and sufficient amount of phytochemicals from unprocessed plant foods, scientists note that cells age more rapidly and do not retain their innate ability to remove and detoxify waste products and toxic compounds. Low levels of phytochemical-rich produce in our modern diet are largely responsible for the common diseases seen with aging. We have learned so much from modern nutritional science in the last 15 years, and when applied to our daily life, it works—we can live longer and better with almost no risk of the diseases that plague most Americans.

Let's take heart disease as an example. Heart attacks are extremely rare occurrences in populations that eat a diet rich in protective phytochemicals (from vegetables) such as the Okinawans of Japan, but are omnipresent in populations, such as ours, that eat a diet low in these protective nutrients.[11] Compelling data from numerous population studies shows that a natural, plant-based diet rich in antioxidants and phytochemicals will prevent, arrest and even reverse heart disease.[12]

Our bodies were designed to make use of thousands of plant compounds. When these necessary compounds are missing, we survive because our bodies are adaptable, but over time we lose our powerful potential for wellness and chronic disease develops. We are robbed of living to our fullest potential in good physical, emotional, and mental health. Consumption of healthy foods leads to disease resistance; consumption of unhealthy foods makes us disease-prone.

Eating right enables you to feel your best every day. You may still get sick from a virus, but your body will be in a far better position to defend itself and make a quick and complete recovery. Optimal nutrition enables us to work better, play better, and maintain our youthful vigor as we age gracefully.

The Health Equation

The secret to a long life and disease reversal is to eat a diet lower in calories but higher in nutrients. It is all about nutrient bang per caloric buck.

This important nutritional concept can be presented by a simple mathematical formula, which I call my health equation.

DR. FUHRMAN'S HEALTH EQUATION:
$$H = N/C$$

Your **H**ealth is dependent on the **N**utrient-per-**C**alorie density of your diet.

In this discussion, the word nutrient means micronutrients. Your future health equals nutrient consumption divided by calories. This straightforward mathematical formula is the basis of nutritional science and nutritional healing. This formula essentially states that for you to be in excellent health, your diet must be nutrient-rich, and you must not overeat on calories (or macronutrients). The nutrient density in your body's tissues is proportional to the nutrient density of your diet.

We realize we must seek out and consume more foods with a high nutrient-per-calorie density and fewer foods with a low nutrient-per-calorie density.[13]

Every nutritional scientist in the world agrees that moderate caloric restriction in the environment of micronutrient adequacy slows the aging process, prevents the development of chronic diseases and extends lifespan. This has been tested in every species of animal, including primates.[14] There is no controversy that Americans are eating themselves to death with too many calories. To change this we must do three things:

1 - EAT LESS FAT
2 - EAT LESS PROTEIN
3 - EAT LESS CARBOHYDRATE

Even though reduction of calories is valuable, the focus here is different. When the fatty foods you eat are high-nutrient fatty foods and the proteins you eat are high-nutrient proteins and the carbohydrates you eat are high-nutrient carbohydrates, you naturally desire fewer calories.

Natural, whole plant foods are a mixture of fat, carbohydrate and protein and in their natural state, they are typically rich in micronutrients.

Simply trying to reduce calories is called dieting, and dieting doesn't work. The reason this program is so successful is because over time, without even trying or noticing it, you will prefer to eat fewer calories. I know that can sound unlikely. Many people think, "Not me," "My body doesn't work that way," or, "It will be a real struggle for me." However, if you follow the plan, it will happen instinctually and almost effortlessly. I have seen it happen to thousands, with all kinds of different backgrounds and eating histories, and I promise, it can happen for you too.

This program will help you achieve superior health and lose weight if you need to, by eating more nutrient-rich foods and fewer high-calorie, low-nutrient foods. **It works because the more high-nutrient food you consume, the less low-nutrient food you desire.**

Foods are nutrient dense when they contain a high level of micronutrients per calorie. Green vegetables win the award for the most nutrient-dense foods on the planet. Therefore, as you move forward in your quest for nutritional excellence, you will eat more and more vegetables. Since they contain the most nutrients per calorie, vegetables have the most powerful association with life-extension and protection from heart disease and cancer.

It is also important to achieve micronutrient diversity. This means obtaining enough of all beneficial nutrients, not merely higher amounts of a select few. Eating a variety of plant foods is the key to achieving micronutrient diversity. Consider mushrooms and onions to illustrate this concept. They may not contain the highest amounts of vitamins and minerals, but they contain a significant amount of protective phytochemicals that are not found in other foods.

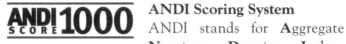 **ANDI Scoring System**

ANDI stands for **A**ggregate **N**utrient **D**ensity **I**ndex. ANDI brings to life the H = N/C health equation or Health = Nutrients divided by Calories. It is an index that guides you on increasing the micronutrient density of your diet. The ANDI Nutrient Score is a rating system that scores foods on a scale of 0–1000. This Index assigns a score to a variety of foods based on adding up most of the vitamins and minerals they deliver for each calorie consumed. The most nutrient dense foods score 1000; all other foods are then scored relative to them. Kale, a dark leafy green, scores 1000 while Coke scores 1. This is just an easy way to quickly visualize the relative nutrient value of various foods. It demonstrates the nutrient power of green vegetables.

Using the ANDI is simple. It is meant to encourage you to eat more foods that have high numbers and eat larger amounts of these foods because the higher the number, and the greater percentage of those foods in your diet, the better your health.

Olive oil, for example, scores only 10 because it is high in calories and low in nutrients. It is important to recognize that olive oil, like all other oil, has 120 calories per tablespoon. People sabotage their attempts to lose weight by using too much oil in their diet.

Because phytochemicals are largely unnamed and unmeasured, these ANDI rankings may underestimate the healthful properties of colorful, natural, plant foods compared to processed foods and animal products. One thing we do know about natural foods is that the foods that contain the highest amount of known nutrients are the same foods that contain the most unknown nutrients. Even though these rankings may not consider the phyto-chemical number sufficiently, they are still a reasonable measurement of their content and can be very helpful in giving you an understanding of the value of the food.

Matter of Emphasis
Most health authorities today are in agreement that we should add more servings of healthy fruits and vegetables to our diet. I disagree. Thinking about our diet in this fashion doesn't adequately address the problem. Instead of thinking of adding those protective fruits, vegetables, beans, seeds and nuts to our disease-causing diet, **these foods must be the main focus of the diet itself.** This is what makes the Nutritarian approach different. Once we understand that concept, then we can add a few servings of foods that are not in this category to the diet each week, and use animal products as condiments or small additions to this naturally nutrient-rich diet.

The following chart provides a sample of ANDI scores for a variety of different foods. Please refer to Chapter Seven for additional ANDI values.

SAMPLE NUTRIENT/CALORIE DENSITY SCORES
Aggregate Nutrient Density Index* (ANDI)

Kale	1000	Tomato	186
Collard Greens	1000	Strawberries	182
Mustard Greens	1000	Sweet Potato	181
Watercress	1000	Zucchini	164
Swiss Chard	895	Artichoke	145
Bok Choy	865	Blueberries	132
Spinach	707	Iceberg Lettuce	127
Arugula	604	Grapes	119
Romaine	510	Pomegranates	119
Brussels Sprouts	490	Cantaloupe	118
Carrots	458	Onions	109
Cabbage	434	Flax Seeds	103
Broccoli	340	Orange	98
Cauliflower	315	Edamame	98
Bell Peppers	265	Cucumber	87
Mushrooms	238	Tofu	82
Asparagus	205	Sesame Seeds	74

Lentils	72	Whole Wheat Bread	30
Peaches	65	Almonds	28
Sunflower Seeds	64	Avocado	28
Kidney Beans	64	Brown Rice	28
Green Peas	63	White Potato	28
Cherries	55	Low Fat Plain Yogurt	28
Pineapple	54	Cashews	27
Apple	53	Chicken Breast	24
Mango	53	Ground Beef, 85% lean	21
Peanut Butter	51	Feta Cheese	20
Corn	45	White Bread	17
Pistachio Nuts	37	White Pasta	16
Oatmeal	36	French Fries	12
Shrimp	36	Cheddar Cheese	11
Salmon	34	Apple Juice	11
Eggs	31	Olive Oil	10
Milk, 1%	31	Vanilla Ice Cream	9
Walnuts	30	Corn Chips	7
Bananas	30	Cola	1

CHAPTER FOUR

TOP 25 FOODS

Now that you know the secret formula to health is $H = N/C$ (Health = Nutrients/Calories), it's time to start putting it into practice. There are comprehensive lists of nutrient density scores later in this book. But to make it easy for you to find the very best foods, I've listed my Top 25 Super Foods on the following page.

Green vegetables, beans, onions, mushrooms, berries and nuts and seeds are among my favorite Super Foods. They contain protective phytochemcals and work together to provide us with optimal health and super immunity from disease.

You have the opportunity to earn great health through the food you eat. Include as many of these Super Foods in your diet as you possibly can.

		NUTRIENT SCORE
1.	Collard, Mustard, Turnip Greens	1000
2.	Kale	1000
3.	Watercress	1000
4.	Swiss Chard	895
5.	Bok Choy	865
6.	Cabbage (all varieties)	434 – 715
7.	Spinach	707
8.	Arugula	604
9.	Lettuce (Boston, Romaine, Red & Green Leaf)	367 – 585
10.	Brussels Sprouts	490
11.	Carrots	458
12.	Broccoli	340
13.	Cauliflower	315
14.	Bell Peppers, red and green	207 – 224
15.	Mushrooms	238
16.	Tomatoes	186
17.	Berries (all varieties)	132 – 182
18.	Asparagus	205
19.	Pomegranates	119
20.	Grapes	119
21.	Cantaloupe	118
22.	Onions	109
23.	Beans (all varieties)	43 – 98
24.	Seeds (flax, hemp, chia, sesame, pumpkin, sunflower)	39 – 103
25.	Nuts (all varieties)	21 – 60

CHAPTER FIVE

THREE LEVELS OF SUPERIOR NUTRITION

I have organized my meal plans into three levels of superior nutrition. Based on your health needs and current dietary habits, you can choose between three different diet options: Level One, Two or Three. I would like to see everyone reach at least Level Two, although for many, even Level One will represent a significant improvement.

Use my ANDI scores contained in Chapter Four and Seven of this book to help you choose the most nutrient dense foods. You will find sample menus and healthy recipes in Chapters Eight and Nine of this handbook. High-nutrient density soups, delicious fruit smoothies and healthy dressings and dips are featured in all my meal plans, however this handbook only gives a sample of the valuable information, menus and recipes available in my more comprehensive *Eat for Health* book and at my web site: www.drfuhrman.com.

I have designed three levels, as an aid to direct people to the level of nutritional excellence they need for their individual health conditions. This does not mean a person should not move to a higher level of excellence if they are comfortable doing so.

**Regardless of what level you choose,
take a 28 day Nutritarian Pledge
to follow these cornerstones of healthy eating:**

INCLUDE DAILY:

1) A large salad

2) At least a half-cup serving of
   beans/legumes in soup, salad or a main dish

3) At least 3 fresh fruits

4) At least one ounce of raw nuts
   and seeds

5) At least one large (double-size)
   serving of steamed green vegetables

AVOID:

1) barbequed, processed and cured meats
   and commercial red meat

2) fried foods

3) full-fat dairy (cheese, ice cream,
   butter, whole milk and 2% milk)
   and trans fat (margarine)

4) soft drinks, sugar and artificial
   sweeteners

5) white flour products

The point is to give your body a real chance to change its biochemistry and build up its nutrient stores. You will see how much better your life can be when you are well nourished.

Level 1

Level 1 is appropriate for a person who is healthy, thin, physically fit and exercises regularly. You should have no risk factors such as high blood pressure, high cholesterol or a family history of heart disease, stroke or cancer before the age of 75.

Most Americans do have risk factors or a family history of strokes, heart attacks and cancer, and most Americans are overweight. So most people should only see Level 1 as a temporary stage as they learn about high-nutrient eating and allow their taste buds to acclimate to higher levels of whole natural plant foods.

Level 1 is designed to ease the emotional shock of making profound dietary improvements. It enables people to revamp their diet at a level that is significant, but not overwhelming. Enjoy this new style of eating, allow your taste preferences to change with time and learn some great recipes. You may soon decide to move to a higher level. However, I still recommend that the majority of individuals make the commitment to jump right into the more nutrient-dense Levels 2 or 3 because so many people are significantly overweight and have risk factors that need to be addressed immediately. People in desperate need of a health makeover need to start on Levels 2 or 3.

On Level 1, you eliminate fried foods and substitute fruit-based healthful desserts and whole grains for low nutrient processed snack foods such as salty snacks, candy, ice cream and baked products. Whole grain products like old fashioned oats, wild rice, brown rice, 100 percent whole grain bread and pasta made with 100 percent whole grain or bean flour are used. Bread and pasta made with refined white flour are eliminated.

Your sodium intake will decrease as you begin to make these dietary changes. Processed foods and restaurant foods contribute 77 percent of the sodium people consume. Salt from the saltshaker provides 11 percent and sodium found naturally in food provides the remaining 12 percent.[15]

You also eliminate foods like cheese and butter that are high in saturated fats. Your cooking techniques use only a minimal amount of oil. Most Americans consume over 20 servings of animal products weekly. In Level 1, I recommend only four servings of animal products per week. These animal products are limited to fish, skinless chicken or turkey, eggs or nonfat dairy products.

Level 2

Level 2 builds on the positive changes described in Level 1. In Level 2, animal products are reduced to three servings weekly and vegetables and beans should start to make up an even larger portion of your total caloric intake. When you incorporate more and more nutrient-rich produce in your diet, you automatically increase your intake of antioxidants, phytochemicals, plant fibers, and plant sterols. You lower the glycemic index of your diet and the level of saturated fat, salt and other negative elements without having to think about it. Your ability to appreciate the natural flavors of unprocessed, whole foods will improve with time because you lose your dependence on salt and sugar. Add more beans and nuts to your diet to replace animal products.

Try some of the high-nutrient dressing and dip recipes in Chapter Nine. They use heart healthy nuts and seeds to replace the oils found in traditional dressings and dips.

Level 2 is a reasonable target diet for most people. If you want to lose weight, lower your cholesterol, lower your blood pressure or just live a long and healthy life, this is the level you should adopt.

Level 3

If you suffer from serious medical conditions like diabetes, heart disease, autoimmune disease or just want to optimize the nutrient density of your diet to slow aging and maximize longevity, step up to Level 3. If you suffer from a medical condition that is important to reverse, this is the right prescription for you. If you are on medications and you want to be able to discontinue them as quickly as possible, go for Level 3. It is also the level to chose if you have trouble losing weight, no matter what you do, and want to maximize your results. Level 3 is designed for those who want to reverse serious disease or for healthy people who want to push the envelope of human longevity.

Level 3 is the diet that I use in my medical practice for people who have serious autoimmune diseases; (such as rheumatoid arthritis or lupus), or when someone has life-threatening heart disease (atherosclerosis). I prescribe it for diabetics who need to lower their blood sugars into the normal range, or to get rid of severe migraines. It delivers the highest level of nutrient density.

Level 3 includes a maximum of two servings of animal products weekly and concentrates on high-nutrient density vegetables. Review the Top 25 food list in Chapter 4 and then use the ANDI scores in Chapter 7 to select the most nutrient dense foods possible. Use green smoothies, fresh vegetable juices, healthful soups and lots of greens and raw vegetables to make every calorie count.

At this level, you should consume processed foods only rarely. Keep the use of refined fats and oils to a minimum. Nuts and seeds supply essential fats in a much healthier package, with significant health benefits. The recipes in Chapter 9 provide some ideas for incorporating a variety of nutrient dense foods into your diet.

In the following table, I have listed some of the top foods in the six food categories that should make up 75-80 percent of your diet. These foods get some of the highest ANDI scores. Below each group, the number of servings suggested to achieve Level 1, 2 or 3 is listed. These amounts should not be seen as rigid requirements, but rather as helpful guidelines. Of course there are many other choices in these categories and I encourage you to try them all.

Three Levels of Super Immunity
Recommended Daily Servings of Vegetables, Fruit, Beans & Nuts

COOKED GREEN VEGETABLES

1.5 cups kale

1.5 cups mustard, turnip or collard greens

1.5 cups bok choy

1.5 cups broccoli rabe

1.5 cups Chinese/napa cabbage

1.5 cups spinach

1.5 cups Brussels sprouts

1.5 cups Swiss chard

1.5 cups cabbage

1.5 cups broccoli

LEVEL ONE	LEVEL TWO	LEVEL THREE
1-2 servings	2-3 servings	2-3 servings

RAW GREEN VEGETABLES

3 cups watercress

5 cups spinach

5 cups romaine, Boston, red or green leaf lettuce

5 cups arugula

5 cups mixed baby greens

1.5 cups raw broccoli

1.5 cups cabbage

1.5 cups green pepper

2 cups zucchini

1.5 cups snow peas

LEVEL ONE	LEVEL TWO	LEVEL THREE
1 serving	1-2 servings	2-3 servings

NON-GREEN VEGETABLES

1 cup carrots

6 radishes

1 cup red pepper

2 cups radicchio

1 cup cauliflower

1 tomato

1/2 cup chopped onion or scallions

1/2 cup cooked mushrooms

LEVEL ONE	LEVEL TWO	LEVEL THREE
1 serving	1 serving	1-2 servings

FRUIT

1.5 cups strawberries

1.5 cups raspberries

1.5 cups blueberries

2 plums

1 orange

1.5 cups cantaloupe

2 kiwis

2.5 cups watermelon

1 apple

1.5 cups cherries

LEVEL ONE	LEVEL TWO	LEVEL THREE
3-5 servings	3-5 servings	3-5 servings

BEANS

1/2 - 1 cup lentils	1/2 - 1 cup split peas
1/2 - 1 cup red kidney	1/2 - 1 cup edamame
1/2 - 1 cup adzuki beans	1/2 - 1 cup chickpeas
1/2 - 1 cup black beans	1/2 - 1 cup white beans
1/2 - 1 cup pinto beans	4 oz tofu

LEVEL ONE	LEVEL TWO	LEVEL THREE
1-3 servings	1-3 servings	1-3 servings

NUTS AND SEEDS

1/4 cup sunflower seeds	1/4 cup pecans
2 tablespoons ground flax, hemp or chia seeds	1/4 cup almonds
	1/4 cup walnuts
1/4 cup sesame seeds	1/4 cup cashews
1/4 cup pumpkin seeds	2 tablespoons raw nut butter
1/4 cup pistachios	

LEVEL ONE	LEVEL TWO	LEVEL THREE
1-3 servings*	1-3 servings*	1-3 servings*

The amount of nuts and seeds as well as other foods you consume depends on your caloric requirements. If you are trying to lose weight, limit nuts to one serving daily. If you are thin, want to gain weight or need more calories to fuel your athletic activities, then the number of servings may be increased.

Eating enough healthy food is critical to your success as a Nutritarian. You will find that when you eat enough high-nutrient food, you no longer desire or even have room for the other foods that used to make up the biggest part of your diet. Processed and refined foods offer little in terms of nutrients and phytochemicals. When you eat them, you are literally throwing away valuable nutrients that could have been put to good use by your body.

Overview of the Three Levels
Recommended Amounts

	LEVEL 1	LEVEL 2	LEVEL 3
VEGETABLES raw & cooked 1 serving = 1-1/2 cups cooked or 2 to 5 cups raw	3-4 servings/day	4-6 servings/day	5-7 servings/day
FRUIT 1 serving = about 1-1/2 cups	3-5 servings/day	3-5 servings/day	3-5 servings/day
BEANS 1 serving = 1/2 to 1 cup	1-2 servings/day	1-2 servings/day	1-2 servings/day
NUTS & SEEDS 1 serving = 1 ounce or 1/4 cup	1-3 servings/day	1-3 servings/day ————1 serving/day if trying to lose weight————	1-3 servings/day
WHOLE GRAIN PRODUCTS/POTATOES 1 serving = 1 slice or 1 cup	1-3 servings/day	1-3 servings/day ————1 serving/day if trying to lose weight————	1-2 servings/day
ANIMAL PRODUCTS* 1 serving = 4 ounces	4 servings/week or less	3 servings/week or less	2 servings/week or less
SODIUM	1200 mg/day or less	1200 mg/day or less	1000 mg/day or less
FATS/OILS Substitutes include non dairy spreads without trans or hydrogenated fats	1 tablespoon of olive oil or acceptable substitute/day	1 tablespoon of olive oil or acceptable substitute/day	1-2 tablespoons/week

* Animal Products include: white meat fowl, fish, eggs, low fat dairy. Absolutely no processed meats, cured meats, barbecued meat or full fat dairy.

My book *Eat for Health* contains more information about my Nutritarian Eating Plans and resolving the emotional impediments to dietary change. It features cooking tips, menus and over 150 healthy recipes.

For those requiring aggressive weight loss and immediate uncompromising results, my book *Eat to Live* offers guidance, structure and a six week plan to kick-start your dietary makeover.

CHAPTER SIX

TOP NUTRITARIAN PRINCIPLES

Here is my Top Ten list of Nutritarian principles.

1. **Your body's immune system needs the right foods to allow it to work to its fullest potential.** By changing our diets and combining foods that contain powerful immune-strengthening capabilities, we can achieve incredible health and prevent and even reverse disease. The standard American diet is nutrient deficient. We are eating too many highly processed foods, foods with added sweeteners and animal fats and proteins. At the same time we are not eating enough fruits, vegetables, seeds and beans, which leaves us lacking in hundreds of the most immune-building compounds.

2. **H=N/C — Dr. Fuhrman's Health Equation**—Your long-term health is directly related to the amount of Nutrients you get for each Calorie. The more "nutrient-dense" a food, the more powerful it is. The most nutrient-dense foods are fruits and vegetables, especially dark leafy greens which are the foods missing in most modern diets. Nutrient-dense foods contain vital nutrients, vitamins and minerals essential for preventing disease, boosting immunity, detoxifying the body and delivering permanent weight loss.

3. **Prescription Medications will not solve your health problems.** Heart disease, Type II diabetes, hypertension and many other conditions are directly related to poor dietary habits. The body has an incredible ability to heal itself when properly nourished. For example, even patients on insulin for years can reduce and eventually eliminate medications as they lose weight and become healthy. Superior nutrition is more effective than medications at resolving most medical problems while promoting a pleasurable, longer and more healthy life.

4. **If you want to lose weight — DON'T DIET!** 95% of all weight lost on most popular diets is regained. While many diets may produce short term weight loss, they cannot be maintained and therefore the weight returns. The only proven strategy for permanent weight

loss is to consume sufficient nutrients and fiber for a lifetime of excellent health. This strategy will reduce your cravings for 'junk' food and curb the tendency to overeat. Then you will instinctually eat fewer calories, without the food addictions and cravings that have sabotaged your attempts in the past.

5. **Where's the Beef?** Remember that vegetables, beans and seeds are high in protein, so there is no essential need to have animal products at every meal. In fact, broccoli has about the same amount of protein as steak. Think about it… cows are vegan, as are gorillas and horses. Trying to lose weight or reduce your cholesterol? Think greens for health and for building lean muscle. To maximize our health and longevity, we need to get more protein from nutrient-rich plant sources such as greens, beans, seeds and nuts and less from animal products.

6. **Remember: G-BOMBS** Greens, Beans, Onions, Mushrooms, Berries and Seeds are important foods with powerful immune-strengthening capabilities. Include these super foods in your diet every day.

7. **Watch the Olive Oil!** One tablespoon of olive oil has 120 calories (all oils do). One-quarter cup has 500 calories. Healthy salads are definitely a way of life for people who want to lose weight or improve health. However, many of the benefits of a salad are lost when the calorie count is increased ten-fold with oil. Flavored vinegars,

fruit, nut and seed-based dressings are the way to go. Nuts and seeds, not oil, have shown dramatic protection against heart disease. We need to get more of our fats from these wholesome foods and less from processed oils.

8. **If health came in a bottle — we'd all be healthy!** Natural, whole, plant-based foods are highly complex. It may never be possible to extract the precise symphony of nutrients found in fruits and vegetables and place it in a pill. So don't rely on pills and supplements to get your primary nutrition.

9. **Six-A-Day... Not The Way!** You have probably heard it's better to eat six small meals a day. That is not ideal. You simply will not need to eat that frequently once your body is well nourished with micronutrients. The body can more effectively detoxify and enhance cell repair when not constantly eating and digesting. Eating healthfully removes cravings and reduces the sensations driving us to eat too much and too often. For most people who follow a nutritarian diet-style, eating when truly hungry means eating three meals a day.

10. **Let Your Body Decide!** Nobody wants to hear that they have to give up all their favorite foods like pizza and ice cream. But wouldn't it be nice if over time your body actually preferred healthy foods? The body can change its taste and food preferences. As you consume

larger and larger portions of health-promoting foods, your appetite for low-nutrient foods decreases and you gradually lose your addiction to sugar and fats. You learn to enjoy and prepare gourmet-tasting meals that are nutrient-rich. When this occurs, you have become a Nutritarian!

I realize unhealthy foods can be very appealing and hard to resist. Please be patient with yourself as you start to eat right. As you switch to healthful foods, you will lose your cravings for unhealthful foods. You will learn to eat only when you are truly hungry. Your body will learn to love fresh fruits and vegetables and my healthful recipes because they taste so great and satisfying.

Becoming a Nutritarian is all about having the knowledge and support you need to get back in touch with the natural wisdom of your body.

CHAPTER SEVEN

NUTRIENT DENSITY SCORES

In this chapter, you will find nutrient/calorie-density scores grouped by category based on the Aggregate Nutrient Density Index (ANDI). Knowing which foods are high in nutrient density (and which are low) will make it easier to get the dramatic health benefits of eating more high-nutrient foods. As you look through these lists, you may discover that many of the foods you currently eat provide little or virtually no nutritional value.

NOTE: *Calorie and Sodium data are provided for reference only. They are not related to ANDI scores. ANDI scores provide a relative ranking based on an equal amount of calories.*

	CALORIES	SODIUM	ANDI
VEGETABLES			
Kale, cooked (1.5 cups)	55	45	1000
Mustard Greens (1.5 cups)	32	34	1000
Collard Greens (1.5 cups)	74	46	1000

	CALORIES	SODIUM	ANDI
Turnip Greens (1.5 cups)	43	63	1000
Watercress (3 cups)	11	42	1000
Swiss Chard (1.5 cups)	53	470	895
Bok Choy (1.5 cups)	31	87	865
Kale, raw (1.5 cups)	50	43	778
Napa Cabbage (1.5 cups)	20	18	715
Spinach, cooked (1.5 cups)	62	189	707
Spinach, raw (5 cups)	35	119	705
Arugula, (5 cups)	25	27	604
Lettuce, green leaf (5 cups)	27	50	585
Chicory (5 cups)	33	65	516
Lettuce, romaine (5 cups)	40	19	510
Lettuce, red leaf (5 cups)	22	35	507
Radish (6 items)	4	11	502
Brussels Sprouts (1.5 cups)	84	49	490
Turnips (1.5 cups)	51	37	473
Carrots, cooked (1.5 cups)	82	136	458
Cabbage, cooked (1.5 cups)	52	18	434
Carrots, raw (1.5 cups)	79	132	384
Lettuce, Boston or Bibb (5 cups)	36	14	367
Broccoli Rabe (1.5 cups)	77	131	366
Kohlrabi (1.5 cups)	72	52	352
Dandelion Greens (1.5 cups)	52	69	347
Broccoli, raw (1.5 cups)	46	45	340

	CALORIES	SODIUM	ANDI
Cabbage, raw (1.5 cups)	33	24	332
Cauliflower, raw (1.5 cups)	40	48	315
Rutabaga (1.5 cups)	99	51	296
Broccoli, cooked (1.5 cups)	82	96	294
Cauliflower, cooked (1.5 cups)	43	28	294
Endive (1.5 cups)	13	17	284
Radicchio (2 cups)	18	18	271
Red Bell Pepper, cooked (1.5 cups)	57	4	265
Pumpkin (1.5 cups)	74	4	249
Butternut Squash (1.5 cups)	123	12	241
Mushrooms, brown	24	6	238
Red Bell Pepper, raw (1.5 cups)	69	9	224
Jalapeno Pepper (1 pepper)	4	0	217
Green Hot Chili Pepper (1 pepper)	18	3	216
Green Bell Pepper, raw (1.5 cups)	28	4	207
Asparagus (1.5 cups)	59	38	205
Mushrooms, white (1.5 cups)	65	5	199
Mushrooms, Portobello (1.5 cups)	28	12	193
Tomato, raw (1.5 cups)	49	14	186
Tomato, cooked (1.5 cups)	65	40	185
Sweet Potato (1 large)	162	65	181
Bean Sprouts (1 cup)	31	6	177
Zucchini, cooked (1.5 cups)	41	8	164
Green Bell Pepper, cooked (1.5 cups)	57	4	158

	CALORIES	SODIUM	ANDI
Okra (1.5 cups)	53	14	155
Celery (1 cup)	16	81	151
Mushrooms, maitake (1.5 cups)	33	1	150
Artichoke (1.5 cups)	134	151	145
Zucchini, raw (1 cup)	33	16	142
Hubbard Squash (1 cup)	103	16	142
Leeks (1.5 cups)	48	16	135
Alfalfa Sprouts (1 cup)	8	2	133
Pasilla pepper, dried (4 peppers)	97	25	127
Lettuce, Iceberg (5 cups)	40	29	127
Sun dried Tomato (0.5 cup)	70	67	124
Garlic Clove (2 cloves)	9	1	118
Wakame Seaweed (0.25 cup)	9	174	118
Onions, cooked (0.5 cup)	46	3	109
Onions, raw (0.5 cup)	32	3	107
Snow Peas, raw (1.5 cups)	40	4	106
Bamboo Shoots (1 cup)	25	9	103
Chayote Squash (1.5 cups)	38	4	101
Green Snap Beans, raw (1.5 cups)	47	9	99
Snow Peas, cooked (1.5 cups)	101	10	97
Shallots, raw (3 tablespoons)	22	4	94
Yellow Squash, cooked (1.5 cups)	62	3	92
Yellow Squash, raw (1.5 cups)	36	4	88
Cucumber, (1 item)	45	6	87
Tomatillo (2 items)	22	1	85

	CALORIES	SODIUM	ANDI
Green Snap Beans, cooked (1.5 cups)	66	2	81
Beets, raw (1.5 cups)	88	159	80
Celeriac (1.5 cups)	63	142	78
Green Peas (1.5 cups)	202	7	63
Beets, cooked (1.5 cups)	112	196	57
Ginger Root (2 teaspoons)	3	1	56
Corn, yellow (1.5 cups)	215	2	45
Jicama (1.5 cups)	74	8	44
Spaghetti Squash (1.5 cups)	63	42	44
Acorn Squash (1.5 cups)	172	12	44
Corn, white (1.5 cups)	228	7	41
Lotus Root (1.5 cups)	79	54	39
Parsnips (1.5 cups)	166	23	37
Water Chestnuts (1.5 cups)	120	17	32
Eggplant (1.5 cups)	52	1	31
Yams (1.5 cups)	237	16	29
White Potato (1.5 cups)	145	8	28
Olives (4 items)	27	244	26
Cassava Root (yucca) (1 cup)	330	29	13
French Fries (20 pieces)	229	540	12

HERBS

Basil (0.25 cup)	1	0	518
Cilantro (0.25 cup)	1	2	481
Parsley (0.25 cup)	5	8	381
Chives (0.25 cup)	3	0	319

	CALORIES	SODIUM	ANDI
FRUIT			
Cranberry, fresh (0.5 cup)	23	1	207
Strawberries (1.5 cups)	80	2	182
Blackberries (1.5 cups)	93	2	171
Raspberries (1.5 cups)	96	2	133
Lemon Juice (2 tablespoons)	5	0	133
Blueberries (1.5 cups)	127	2	132
Guava (1 item)	37	1	125
Grapefruit (1.5 cups)	110	0	120
Pomegranates (1 item)	234	8	119
Grapes (1.5 cups)	156	5	119
Cantaloupe (1.5 cups)	82	38	118
Lime Juice (2 tablespoons)	11	1	117
Plums (1.5 cups)	114	0	106
Orange (1 item)	86	0	98
Tangerine (1.5 cups)	155	6	86
Apricots, fresh (1.5 cups)	67	1	75
Watermelon, (2.5 cups)	114	4	71
Papaya (1.5 cups)	94	17	69
Peaches (1 item)	68	0	65
Kiwi (2 items)	84	4	61
Figs, fresh (3 items)	111	2	56
Cherries (1.5 cups)	130	0	55
Persimmons (1 item)	118	2	54

	CALORIES	SODIUM	ANDI
Pineapple (1.5 cups)	124	2	54
Mango (1.5 cups)	149	2	53
Apples (I item)	116	2	53
Kumquats (7 items)	94	13	51
Passion Fruit (1 cup)	229	66	44
Cranberries, dried sweetened (0.25 cup)	93	1	42
Pears (1 item)	133	2	40
Nectarine (1 item)	69	0	39
Cherimoya (1 item)	176	16	38
Honeydew Melon (1.5 cups)	92	46	31
Banana (1 item)	121	1	30
Avocado (0.5 item)	114	5	28
Apricots, dried (0.25 cup)	78	3	26
Currants, dried (0.25 cup)	102	3	21
Figs, dried (0.25 cup)	63	3	21
Dates, diglet noor (4 dates)	80	1	17
Tamarind (0.5 cup)	143	17	16
Dates, medjool (2 dates)	133	1	15
Raisins (0.25 cup)	108	4	15
Coconut, dried, unsweetened (1 cup)	122	7	10
Applesauce, unsweetened (1 cup)	102	5	9
Applesauce, sweetened (1 cup)	167	5	6

	CALORIES	SODIUM	ANDI

FRUIT/VEGETABLE JUICES

	CALORIES	SODIUM	ANDI
Carrot Juice (1 cup)	94	156	446
Vegetable Juice (1 cup)	46	480	284
Tomato Juice, no-salt-added (1 cup)	41	24	225
Tomato Juice, regular (1 cup)	41	654	225
Pomegranate Juice (1 cup)	134	22	102
Coconut Water (1 cup)	46	252	83
Grapefruit Juice (1 cup)	96	2	48
Orange Juice (1 cup)	112	2	46
Grape Juice (1 cup)	152	13	45
Prune Juice (1 cup)	182	10	33
Cranberry Juice Cocktail (1 cup)	137	5	32
Pineapple Juice (1 cup)	133	5	21
Coconut Milk (1 cup)	552	36	14
Apple Juice (1 cup)	114	10	11

BEANS/LEGUMES

	CALORIES	SODIUM	ANDI
Edamame (1 cup)	189	9	98
Pinto Beans (1 cup)	245	2	86
Tofu (1 cup)	365	35	82
Great Northern Beans (1 cup)	209	4	77
Adzuki Beans (1 cup)	294	18	74
Lentils (1 cup)	230	4	72
Lima Beans (1 cup)	216	4	69
Tempeh (4 ounces)	320	15	66
Kidney Beans (1 cup)	225	2	64

	CALORIES	SODIUM	ANDI
Black Beans (1 cup)	227	2	61
Chickpeas (1 cup)	269	11	55
Split Peas (1 cup)	231	4	43
Hummus (0.5 cup)	218	298	21

NUTS AND SEEDS

NUTS

Peanuts, unsalted (0.25 cup)	214	2	59
Pistachio Nuts, unsalted (0.25 cup)	173	0	37
Chestnuts (1 ounce)	56	1	34
Hazelnuts (1 ounce)	218	0	34
Pecans (1 ounce)	188	0	33
Walnuts (0.25 cup)	191	1	30
Pine Nuts (0.25 cup)	227	1	28
Almonds, unsalted (0.25 cup)	214	7	28
Cashews, unsalted (0.25 cup)	197	5	27
Brazil Nuts (0.25 cup)	218	1	26
Macadamia Nuts, unsalted (0.25 cup)	203	4	21

SEEDS

Flax Seeds (2 tablespoons)	110	6	103
Chia Seeds (2 tablespoons)	146	5	77
Sesame Seeds, unhulled (2 tablespoons)	103	2	74
Hemp Seeds (2 tablespoons)	174	5	65
Sunflower Seeds (0.25 cup)	204	3	64
Sesame Seeds, hulled (2 tablespoons)	101	8	56
Pumpkin Seeds (0.25 cup)	180	2	39

	CALORIES	SODIUM	ANDI
NUT AND SEED BUTTER			
Tahini (2 tablespoons)	179	35	60
Sunflower Seed Butter (2 tablespoons)	197	1	55
Peanut Butter, no-salt-added (2 tbsp)	197	5	51
Almond Butter, no-salt-added (2 tbsp)	196	2	29
Cashew Butter, no-salt-added (2 tbsp)	188	5	26

GRAINS

WHOLE GRAINS			
Black Rice, cooked (1 cup)	218	8	96
Wild Rice, cooked (1 cup)	166	5	56
Oats, old fashioned, cooked (1 cup)	166	9	36
Bulgur, cooked (1 cup)	151	9	33
Buckwheat groats, cooked (1 cup)	155	7	30
Quinoa, cooked (1 cup)	222	13	28
Brown Rice, cooked (1 cup)	216	10	28
Kamut, cooked (1 cup)	251	10	27
Barley, cooked (1 cup)	193	5	24
Millet, cooked (1 cup)	207	3	23
Cornmeal (0.24 cup)	110	11	17

REFINED GRAINS (see note regarding fortification on page 77)			
Wheat flour, whole wheat (0.25 cup)	102	1	31
Pasta, whole wheat (1 cup cooked)	174	4	25
Estimated ANDI without fortification			*22*

	CALORIES	SODIUM	ANDI
Pasta, spinach (1 cup cooked)	182	20	24
Pasta, white (1 cup cooked)	221	1	16
Estimated ANDI without fortification			*11*
Barley, pearled (1 cup cooked)	193	5	15
White Rice (1 cup cooked)	205	2	13
Estimated ANDI without fortification			*8*
Couscous (1 cup cooked)	176	8	13
Estimated ANDI without fortification			*10*
Wheat flour, white (0.25 cup)	114	1	8
Estimated ANDI without fortification			*6*

BREADS AND CRACKERS *(see note regarding fortification on page 77)*

Bread, whole wheat (1 slice)	69	132	30
English Muffin, whole wheat (1 muffin)	134	240	29
Pita, whole wheat (1 large)	170	340	26
Pumpernickel Bread (1 slice)	65	174	25
Estimated ANDI without fortification			*18*
Bagel, whole wheat (1 bagel)	245	430	19
Bread, white (1 slice)	74	137	17
Estimated ANDI without fortification			*9*
Pita, white (1 large)	165	322	16
Estimated ANDI without fortification			*8*
Melba Toast Crackers (4 pieces)	78	120	15
Estimated ANDI without fortification			*10*
Raisin Bread (1 slice)	71	39	15
Estimated ANDI without fortification			*8*
Tortilla, corn (2 medium)	115	6	13

	CALORIES	SODIUM	ANDI
Tortilla, flour (2 medium)	208	306	13
Estimated ANDI without fortification			7
Sandwich Crackers/peanut butter filling (4 crackers)	138	252	13
Estimated ANDI without fortification			9
English Muffin (1 muffin)	134	264	13
Estimated ANDI without fortification			5
Bagel, plain (1 bagel)	289	561	12
Estimated ANDI without fortification			5
Rice Cake Cracker (4 inch piece)	66	12	12
Saltines (5 crackers)	63	167	11
Estimated ANDI without fortification			5
Sandwich Crackers/cheese filling(4 crackers)	134	249	10
Estimated ANDI without fortification			6

CEREALS *(see note regarding fortification on page 77)*

	CALORIES	SODIUM	ANDI
Bran Flakes Cereal (1 cup)	128	293	67
Estimated ANDI without fortification			26
Corn Flakes Cereal (1 cup)	102	202	54
Estimated ANDI without fortification			3
Granola (1 cup)	429	51	16
Estimated ANDI without fortification			8

FISH

FRESH

	CALORIES	SODIUM	ANDI
Tuna* (4 ounces)	147	61	47
Salmon (4 ounces)	191	152	34

	CALORIES	SODIUM	ANDI
Haddock (4 ounces)	102	296	33
Swordfish** (4 ounces	195	110	30
Cod (4 ounces)	119	88	28
Flounder or Sole (4 ounces)	97	411	27
Tilapia (4 ounces)	143	63	27
Trout, wild (4 ounces)	170	63	25
Red Snapper* (4 ounces)	145	65	25
Grouper* (4 ounces)	134	60	23

CANNED

	CALORIES	SODIUM	ANDI
Anchovy, canned in oil (4 ounces)	238	4159	37
Sardines, canned in oil (4 ounces)	236	573	30
Salmon, canned (4 ounces)	189	462	29
Tuna*, canned in water (4 ounces)	145	427	25

SHELLFISH

	CALORIES	SODIUM	ANDI
Lobster*, boiled (4 ounces)	101	551	67
Blue Crab, boiled (4 ounces)	94	448	60
Alaska King Crab, boiled (4 ounces)	110	1215	55
Shrimp, boiled (4 ounces)	135	1073	36

Fish and shellfish may contain mercury and other pollutants [16]
*** High level of mercury/pollutants*
** Intermediate level of mercury/pollutants*

	CALORIES	SODIUM	ANDI

MEAT

BEEF *(broiled)*

	CALORIES	SODIUM	ANDI
Flank Steak, separable lean and fat, 0" fat (4 ounces)	229	60	26
Skirt Steak, separable lean and fat, 0" fat (4 ounces)	232	86	24
Ground Beef, 90% lean (4 ounces)	178	56	24
Top Round, separable lean and fat, 1/8" fat (4 ounces)	254	45	23
Ground Beef, 85% lean (4 ounces)	284	82	21
Top Sirloin, separable lean and fat, 1/8" fat (4 ounces)	291	61	20
New York Strip, separable lean and fat, 1/8" fat (4 ounces)	299	61	19
Tenderloin, separable lean and fat, 1/8" fat (4 ounces)	303	61	19
Rib Eye, separable lean and fat, 1/8" fat (4 ounces)	301	60	18
Porterhouse, separable lean and fat, 1/8" fat (4 ounces)	337	73	16
Prime Rib, separable lean and fat, 1/8" fat, (4 ounces)	399	71	14

VEAL

	CALORIES	SODIUM	ANDI
Veal Scaloppini/Veal Leg/Cutlets, top round, roasted (4 ounces)	181	77	29
Ground Veal, broiled (4 ounces)	195	94	27

	CALORIES	SODIUM	ANDI
Veal Shank, braised (4 ounces)	216	105	26
Veal Chops, roasted (4 ounces)	258	104	18

Bison

	CALORIES	SODIUM	ANDI
Bison, round steak, broiled (4 ounces)	166	46	37
Bison, ground, broiled (4 ounces)	203	86	32

Lamb

	CALORIES	SODIUM	ANDI
Lamb, Leg, separable lean & fat, 1/8" fat, roasted (4 ounces)	274	76	21
Ground Lamb, broiled (4 ounces)	321	92	20
Lamb, Loin Chops, separable lean & fat, ¼" fat, broiled (4 ounces)	358	87	17

Pork

	CALORIES	SODIUM	ANDI
Pork Tenderloin, separable lean & fat, broiled (4 ounces)	228	73	29
Pork Chops, bone-in, separable lean & fat, broiled (4 ounces)	252	98	27
Pork Chops, boneless, separable lean & fat, broiled (4 ounces)	229	66	27
Pork Loin, separable lean & fat, broiled (4 ounces)	274	70	23
Ham, cured, separable lean & fat, roasted (4 ounces)	275	1345	17
Pork Spareribs, separable lean & fat, braised (4 ounces)	450	105	14
Bacon, broiled or pan fried (2 ounces)	307	1310	13

	CALORIES	SODIUM	ANDI
POULTRY			
Ground Turkey, 93% lean, broiled (4 ounces)	235	103	26
Turkey breast, roasted (4 ounces)	178	73	24
Turkey, dark meat, roasted (4 ounces)	213	90	24
Chicken breast, roasted (4 ounces)	196	87	24
Chicken, dark meat, roasted (4 ounces)	232	105	18
Chicken nuggets, cooked (4 ounces)	336	632	11
Turkey bacon, cooked (2 ounces)	214	1280	10
COLD CUTS			
Roast Beef (2 ounces)	92	21	29
Turkey, deli cut (2 ounces)	64	682	27
Ham, 11% fat (2 ounces)	92	739	26
Bologna, beef and pork (2 ounces)	175	544	13
HOT DOGS AND SAUSAGE			
Italian Turkey Sausage (4 ounces)	179	1052	28
Bratwurst (4 ounces)	378	959	15
Turkey Hot Dog (1 item)	100	485	14
Italian Pork Sausage (4 ounces)	390	1369	13
Pepperoni (2 ounces)	277	926	12
Kielbasa (4 ounces)	350	1025	12
Beef and Pork Hot Dog (1 item)	137	504	10
Breakfast Sausage (4 ounces)	363	1034	7

	CALORIES	SODIUM	ANDI

DAIRY PRODUCTS & EGGS

Beverages

Milk, skim (1 cup)	83	103	38
Milk, 1% fat (1 cup)	102	107	31
Buttermilk (1 cup)	98	257	26
Milk, whole, 3.3% fat (1 cup)	149	105	22
Chocolate Milk, reduced fat (1 cup)	190	165	21
Half & Half (2 tablespoons)	22	7	5
Heavy Whipping Cream (2 tablespoons)	104	11	5

Cheese

Cottage Cheese, low fat (1 cup)	163	918	21
Feta Cheese (2 ounces)	150	633	20
Swiss Cheese (2 ounces)	215	109	16
Cottage Cheese (1 cup)	206	764	16
Ricotta, part skim (0.5 cup)	170	154	16
Mozzarella, part skim (2 ounces)	144	351	15
Goat Cheese (2 ounces)	152	209	15
Mozzarella, whole milk (2 ounces)	170	356	15
American Cheese (1 slice; 1 ounce)	104	468	14
Parmesan (1 ounce)	111	454	14
Blue Cheese (2 ounces)	200	791	13
Provolone (2 ounces)	199	497	13
Gouda (2 ounces)	202	46	13
Brie (2 ounces)	189	357	12

	CALORIES	SODIUM	ANDI
Muenster (2 ounces)	209	356	12
Ricotta, whole milk (0.5 cup)	214	103	12
Cream Cheese, low fat (2 ounces)	115	268	11
Cheddar Cheese (2 ounces)	229	352	11
Neufchatel (2 ounces)	143	189	7
Cream Cheese (2 ounces)	194	182	6

EGGS

	CALORIES	SODIUM	ANDI
Eggs, cooked (1 item)	78	62	31

YOGURT

	CALORIES	SODIUM	ANDI
Tofu Yogurt (1 cup)	246	92	44
Plain Yogurt, fat free (1 cup)	137	189	33
Plain Yogurt, low fat (1 cup)	154	171	28
Fruit Yogurt, low fat (1 cup)	250	142	16
Fruit Yogurt, fat free (1 cup)	233	142	15

NON DAIRY MILK

	CALORIES	SODIUM	ANDI
Soy Milk, original and vanilla with added calcium, vitamin A and D (1 cup)	104	114	37
Soy Milk, original and vanilla, unfortified (1 cup)	131	124	25

PREPARED FOODS

CANNED FOODS

	CALORIES	SODIUM	ANDI
Pumpkin (0.5 cup)	42	6	471
Tomato Sauce (0.25 cup)	15	321	244

	CALORIES	SODIUM	ANDI
Tomato Sauce, no-salt-added (0.25 cup)	18	7	207
Tomato Paste, no-salt-added (2 tbsp)	26	19	174
Tomato Paste (2 tbsp)	27	259	174
Tomatoes, packed in tomato sauce (1 cup)	41	343	153
Green Peas, no-salt-added (1.5 cups)	131	22	70
Green Peas, (1.5 cups)	144	459	64
Peaches, in own juice (1.5 cups)	165	15	45
Peaches, in light syrup (1.5 cups)	203	19	36
Peaches, in heavy syrup (1.5 cups)	291	24	26
Corn, whole kernel (1 cup)	164	545	24
Corn, whole kernel, no-salt-added (1 cup)	164	31	23
Corn, cream style (1 cup)	184	730	21

FAST FOODS *(see note regarding fortification on page 77)*

	CALORIES	SODIUM	ANDI
Egg, Ham and Cheese Muffin (1 item)	299	860	17
Estimated ANDI without fortification			*15*
Cheese Pizza (2 slices)	483	1354	15
Estimated ANDI without fortification			*12*
Fast Food Hamburger (1 item)	265	532	12
Estimated ANDI without fortification			*9*
Fast Food Chicken Sandwich (1 item)	524	1178	12
Estimated ANDI without fortification			*11*
Fast Food Cheeseburger (1 item)	313	745	12
Estimated ANDI without fortification			*9*
Bacon, Egg and Cheese Biscuit (1 item)	432	1225	11
Estimated ANDI without fortification			*9*
Fast Food Milk Shake, vanilla (12 fl oz)	419	142	10

	CALORIES	SODIUM	ANDI
Fast Food French Fries (1 medium serving)	370	266	9
Fast Food Fish Sandwich (1 item)	391	689	8
Estimated ANDI without fortification			*6*

FROZEN DESSERTS

Frozen Yogurt, vanilla (1 cup)	141	110	18
Ice Cream, vanilla (1 cup)	273	106	9
Frozen Fruit and Juice Bar (1 item)	80	4	6
Ice Cream Bar/Stick, chocolate covered (1 item)	166	34	6
Sherbet, fruit (1 cup)	213	68	6
Ice Cream Cookie Sandwich (1 item)	197	133	5

SNACKS (see note regarding fortification on page 77)

Dark Chocolate, 45-59% cocoa solids (1.5 ounces)	232	10	33
Dark Chocolate, 60-69% cocoa solids (1.5 ounces)	246	4	32
Soy Chips or Crisps (1 ounce)	109	239	28
Milk Chocolate, (1.5 ounces)	235	35	16
Rice Crispy Bar (1 bar; 1 ounce)	113	78	16
Estimated ANDI without fortification			*7*
Pretzels, hard, whole wheat (1 ounce)	103	58	15
Popcorn, air popped (4 cups)	124	3	14
Pita Chips (1 ounce)	128	239	14
Estimated ANDI without fortification			*8*

	CALORIES	SODIUM	ANDI
Bagel Chips (1 ounce)	128	66	14
Estimated ANDI without fortification			*6*
Potato Chips (1 ounce)	154	136	13
Beef Jerky (1 piece)	82	416	13
Pretzels, hard (1 ounce)	108	385	12
Estimated ANDI without fortification			*5*
Potato Chips, reduced fat, no salt (1 ounce)	138	2	12
Chocolate Chip Granola Bars (1 bar)	105	83	9
Graham Crackers (2 crackers)	59	67	8
Estimated ANDI without fortification			*5*
Chocolate Sandwich Cookie (2 cookies)	108	116	8
Estimated ANDI without fortification			*5*
Fig Bars (2 cookies)	111	112	8
Estimated ANDI without fortification			*5*
Oatmeal Cookies (2 cookies)	162	138	7
Estimated ANDI without fortification			*5*
Fruit Snacks (0.75 ounce)	75	85	7
Animal Crackers (10 crackers)	112	121	7
Estimated ANDI without fortification			*3*
Corn chips (1 ounce)	147	155	7
Banana Chips (1 ounce)	147	2	7
Corn Puffs (1 ounce)	160	258	6
Peanut Butter Cookie (2 cookies)	143	125	6
Estimated ANDI without fortification			*4*
Popcorn, oil popped microwave (4 cups)	257	466	6

	CALORIES	SODIUM	ANDI
Chocolate Chip Cookies (2 cookies)	95	69	6
Estimated ANDI without fortification			*4*
Chocolate Cake with frosting (1 piece; 1/12 of a cake)	537	480	6
Estimated ANDI without fortification			*5*
Pound Cake (1 piece;1/10 of a cake)	116	119	6
Estimated ANDI without fortification			*3*
Tortilla Chips, nacho cheese (1 ounce)	146	174	5
Apple Pie (1 piece; 1/8 of a pie)	296	251	4

OTHER

BEVERAGES

Red Wine (4 ounces)	100	5	30
White Wine (4 ounces)	96	6	7
Beer (12 ounces)	153	14	7
Cola (8 ounces)	91	10	1

SPREADS/DIPS

Jam/Preserves (1 tablespoon)	56	6	4
Butter (1 tablespoon)	102	101	3
Jelly (1 tablespoon)	56	6	2

	CALORIES	SODIUM	ANDI
Sweeteners			
Maple Syrup (2 tablespoons)	104	5	15
Brown Sugar (1 tablespoon)	34	3	1
Corn Syrup (2 tablespoons)	125	27	1
White Sugar (1 tablespoon)	49	0	0
Oils			
Olive Oil (1 tablespoon)	119	0	10
Sunflower Oil (1 tablespoon)	120	0	8
Corn/Canola Oil (1 tablespoon)	124	0	2
Vinegars			
Balsamic Vinegar (1 tablespoon)	14	4	4

Note: Many processed foods in the Refined Grains, Breads & Crackers, Cereals, Fast Foods and Snacks categories are enriched or fortified with B-complex vitamins, iron and other nutrients. Enrichment and fortification put back only a small percentage of the hundreds of valuable health-promoting components lost during processing. Processing and refining also create unhealthy compounds not found in whole natural foods.

In my ANDI scores for processed, refined foods, I have included estimates of what the ANDI would be without artificial enrichment or fortification. This gives you a more accurate picture of the insignificant nutritional value of these foods.

Appendix: How the ANDI was calculated

To determine the ANDI scores, an equal-calorie serving of each food was evaluated. The following nutrients were included in the evaluation: fiber, calcium, iron, magnesium, phosphorus, potassium, zinc, copper, manganese, selenium, vitamin A, beta carotene, alpha carotene, lycopene, lutein and zeaxanthin, vitamin E, vitamin C, thiamin, riboflavin, niacin, pantothenic acid, vitamin B6, folate, vitamin B12, choline, vitamin K, phytosterols, glucosinolates, angiogenesis inhibitors, organosulfides, aromatase inhibitors, resistant starch, resveratrol plus ORAC score. ORAC (Oxygen Radical Absorbance Capacity) is a measure of the antioxidant or radical scavenging capacity of a food. For consistency, nutrient quantities were converted from their typical measurement conventions (mg, mcg, IU) to a percentage of their Dietary Reference Intake (DRI). For nutrients that have no DRI, goals were established based on available research and current understanding of the benefits of these factors.

To make it easier to compare foods, the raw point totals were converted (multiplied by the same number) so that the highest ranking foods (leafy green vegetables such as mustard greens, kale and collards) received a score of 1000, and the other foods received lower scores accordingly

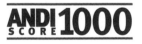

Please note: I am not claiming that ANDI is the only factor to consider when devising the proper diet. However, it is likely the most important factor. There are other scoring systems proposed and in use. The concern here is bias, results influenced by social, economic, or dietary agendas and preferences and not purely by science. In contrast, every effort was made to assure that ANDI is simply a mathematical formula that scores positive elements in food using dependable data, comprehensively, but without any preconceived or other promotional agenda. The results are mathematical and scientific, not opinion derived.

CHAPTER EIGHT

HIGH-NUTRIENT MENUS

Earlier, we discussed my three levels of nutritional excellence. In this chapter, we will do a comparison between a sample menu for each of the three levels against the Standard American Diet.

All items with an asterisk appear in Chapter 9, High-nutrient Recipes, beginning on page 87.

LEVEL ONE

Standard American Diet	Nutritarian Diet
BREAKFAST	BREAKFAST
Orange juice	Fresh squeezed orange juice
Cheerios	Cinnamon Fruit Oatmeal*
Whole milk	
LUNCH	LUNCH
Ham & cheese sandwich on roll w/ mayo	Turkey sandwich on whole grain bread w/ mixed greens & tomato
Potato chips	Strawberries
Coke	Water
DINNER	DINNER
Crackers w/ cheese spread	Tasty Hummus w/ raw veggies*
Spaghetti and meatballs	Pasta w/ Roasted Vegetables*
Vanilla ice cream	Creamy Banana Walnut Ice Cream*

these items appear in Chapter 9, High-nutrient Recipes, beginning on page 87.

Nutritional Analysis	SAD	Nutritarian
Calories	2011	1942
Protein (g)	78	71
Carbohydrate (g)	249	382
Fat (g)	84	29
Cholesterol (mg)	337	20
Saturated fat (g)	38	4
Fiber (g)	15	54
Sodium (mg)	3660	1582
Vitamin C (mg)	183	603
B1, thiamine (mg)	2	3
B6, pyridoxine (mg)	1	3
Iron (mg)	23	23
Folate (mg)	409	802
Magnesium (mg)	148	491
Calcium (mg)	890	681
Zinc (mg)	9	9
Selenium (mcg)	89	122
Alpha tocopherol (mcg)	3	8
Beta carotene (mcg)	120	10,339
Alpha Carotene (mcg)	15	2,782
Lutein & Zeaxanthin (mcg)	300	1,310
Lycopene (mcg)	0	3,532
TOTAL NUTRIENT SCORE	**26**	**55**

LEVEL TWO

Standard American Diet	Nutritarian Diet
BREAKFAST	BREAKFAST
Blueberry muffin	Chocolate Cherry Smoothie*
Coffee/cream	
LUNCH	LUNCH
Nachos w/ cheese	Bean Enchiladas*
Cookies	Apple
DINNER	DINNER
Iceberg lettuce salad w/Italian dressing	Mixed greens w/ Orange Sesame Dressing*
Fried chicken	Creole Chicken with Broccoli and Spinach*
French fries	Brown Rice
Corn	Berry Cobbler*
Cake	

*these items appear
in Chapter 9, High-
nutrient Recipes,
beginning on page 87.

Nutritional Analysis	SAD	Nutritarian
Calories	2030	1830
Protein (g)	81	77
Carbohydrate (g)	217	340
Fat (g)	96	34
Cholesterol (mg)	277	72
Saturated fat (g)	32	6
Fiber (g)	15	62
Sodium (mg)	2889	440
Vitamin C (mg)	42	396
B1, thiamine (mg)	1	2
B6, pyridoxine (mg)	1	4
Iron (mg)	9	21
Folate (mg)	255	1199
Magnesium (mg)	215	742
Calcium (mg)	746	876
Zinc (mg)	8	10
Selenium (mcg)	59	139
Alpha tocopherol (mcg)	5	10
Beta carotene (mcg)	786	22,581
Alpha Carotene (mcg)	5	4465
Lutein & Zeaxanthin (mcg)	1257	11,978
Lycopene (mcg)	795	10,471
TOTAL NUTRIENT SCORE	**19**	**71**

LEVEL THREE

Standard American Diet	**Nutritarian Diet**

BREAKFAST

Bagel w/ cream cheese

Orange juice

LUNCH

Bacon ranch salad w/ crispy chicken

Ice tea

DINNER

Chicken noodle soup

Grilled cheese sandwich

Potato salad

Brownie

BREAKFAST

Lettuce, Banana & Cashew Wrap*

Pomegranate juice

LUNCH

Romaine & spinach salad w/ Almond Balsamic Vinaigrette Dressing*

Fresh fruit & nut bowl

DINNER

Raw veggies w/ Island Black Dip*

Dr. Fuhrman's Famous Anti-Cancer Soup*

Banana Oat Bars*

* these items appear
  in Chapter 9, High-
  nutrient Recipes,
  beginning on page 87.

Nutritional Analysis	SAD	Nutritarian
Calories	2028	1985
Protein (g)	67	70
Carbohydrate (g)	212	335
Fat (g)	105	58
Cholesterol (mg)	283	.2
Saturated fat (g)	32	10
Fiber (g)	11	62
Sodium (mg)	3832	1123
Vitamin C (mg)	167	495
B1, thiamine (mg)	1	2
B6, pyridoxine (mg)	.5	3
Iron (mg)	12	23
Folate (mg)	474	916
Magnesium (mg)	129	642
Calcium (mg)	569	517
Zinc (mg)	5	10
Selenium (mcg)	62	129
Alpha tocopherol (mcg)	3	10
Beta carotene (mcg)	1,557	36,165
Alpha Carotene (mcg)	.02	6,089
Lutein & Zeaxanthin (mcg)	.4	64,395
Lycopene (mcg)	0	3,167
TOTAL NUTRIENT SCORE	19	91

CHAPTER NINE

HIGH-NUTRIENT RECIPES

High-nutrient recipes taste great and are good for you! Those that follow are among the most healthful recipes in the world. Enjoy them, create variations, and start on the road to your optimal weight and health. In addition to the recipes in this book, you can find many more delightful high-nutrient recipes on my website (www.DrFuhrman.com). The member center at drfuhrman.com has over one thousand recipes which are rated and commented on by members.

BREAKFASTS

CHOCOLATE CHERRY SMOOTHIE   *Serves 2*

4 ounces organic baby spinach

1/2 cup unsweetened soy, hemp or almond milk

1/2 cup regular or cherry pomegranate juice

1 tablespoon natural cocoa powder

1 cup frozen cherries

1 banana

1 cup frozen blueberries

1/2 teaspoon vanilla extract

2 tablespoons ground flax seeds

In a high-powered blender, liquefy the spinach with soy milk and juice. Add remaining ingredients and blend about 2 minutes until very smooth.

Per Serving:
Calories 259; Protein 6 g; Carbohydrate 52 g; Total Fat 5 g;
Saturated Fat 0.8 g; Sodium 75 mg

CINNAMON FRUIT OATMEAL   *Serves: 2*

1 cup water
1 teaspoon vanilla extract
1/4 teaspoon cinnamon
1/2 cup old-fashioned rolled oats
1/2 cup blueberries
2 apples, chopped
2 tablespoons chopped walnuts
1 tablespoon ground flax seeds
1/4 cup raisins

In a saucepan, combine water with the vanilla and cinnamon. Bring to a boil over high heat. Reduce the heat to a simmer and stir in the oats.

When the mixture starts to simmer, add the blueberries. Remove from heat when berries are heated through.

Cover and let stand for 15 minutes until thick and creamy.

Mix in apples, nuts, flax seeds, and raisins.

Per Serving:
Calories 241; Protein 13g; Carbohydrates 41g; Total Fat 8.1g;
Saturated Fat 0.8g; Sodium 7mg

BANANA CASHEW LETTUCE WRAP   *Serves 2*

1/4 cup raw cashew butter

12 romaine lettuce leaves

2 bananas, thinly sliced

Spread about 1 teaspoon cashew butter on each lettuce leaf. Lay a few banana slices on the cashew butter and roll up like a burrito.

Per Serving:
Calories 312; Protein 8 g; Carbohydrate 39 g; Total Fat 17 g;
Saturated Fat 3 g; Sodium 15 g

BANANA OAT BARS   *Serves 8*

2 cups quick-cooking rolled oats (not instant)

1/4 cup chopped walnuts

1/2 cup shredded coconut

1/2 cup raisins or chopped dates

2 large ripe bananas, mashed

3/4 cup finely chopped apple

Preheat oven to 350 degrees. Mix ingredients in a large bowl until well combined. Press into a 9" X 9" baking pan. Bake for 30 minutes. Cool on wire rack. When cool, slice into squares or bars.

Can be served for breakfast or as a healthy dessert.

Per Serving:
Calories 250; Protein 8 g; Carbohydrate 42 g; Total Fat 7 g;
Saturated Fat 2 g; Sodium 3 g

SOUPS AND STEWS

Creamy Zucchini Soup   *Serves 4*

1 large onion, chopped

3 cloves garlic, chopped

2 pounds zucchini (about 5 medium), chopped

1 teaspoon dried basil

1/2 teaspoon dried thyme

1/2 teaspoon dried oregano

4 cups low sodium or no-salt-added vegetable broth

1/4 cup raw cashews or 1/8 cup raw cashew butter

4 cups baby spinach

2 cups corn kernels*

1/4 teaspoon black pepper or to taste

Add onion, garlic, zucchini, basil, thyme, oregano and vegetable broth to a large soup pot. Bring to a boil, reduce heat and simmer for 25 minutes or until zucchini is tender.

Pour into a food processor or high-powered blender (in batches, if necessary), add the cashews and blend until smooth and creamy.

Return soup to the pot, add corn and baby spinach, bring to a simmer and cook until spinach is wilted. Add water if needed to adjust consistency. Season with black pepper.

* *Use fresh or defrosted frozen corn kernels. If using fresh corn, boil 2 ears of corn until tender, about 4 minutes. Cut kernels from cobs with a sharp knife.*

Per Serving
Calories 195; Protein 10g; Carbohydrates 33g; Total Fat 5.4g;
Saturated Fat 1.1g; Sodium 431mg

DR. FUHRMAN'S FAMOUS ANTI-CANCER SOUP   *Serves 10*

1 cup dried split peas and/or beans

4 cups water

6-10 medium zucchini

5 pounds carrots, juiced (5-6 cups juice; see note)*

2 bunches celery, juiced (2 cups juice; see note)*

2 tablespoons Dr. Fuhrman's VegiZest or other no-salt seasoning, adjusted to taste

1 teaspoon Mrs. Dash no-salt seasoning

4 medium onions, chopped

3 leek stalks, coarsely chopped

2 bunches kale, collard greens or other greens, tough stems and center ribs removed and leaves chopped

1 cup raw cashews

2 1/2 cups fresh mushrooms (shiitake, cremini and/or white), chopped

Place the beans and water in a very large pot over low heat. Bring to a boil, reduce heat and simmer. Add the zucchini whole to the pot. Add the carrot juice, celery juice, VegiZest and Mrs. Dash.

Put the onions, leeks and kale in a blender and blend with a little bit of the soup liquid. Pour this mixture into the soup pot.

Remove the softened zucchini with tongs and blend them in the blender with the cashews until creamy. Pour this mixture back into the soup pot. Add the mushrooms and continue to simmer the beans until soft, about 2 hours total cooking time.

* *Freshly juiced organic carrots and celery will maximize the flavor of this soup.*

Per Serving:
Calories 304; Protein 14 g; Carbohydrate 52 g; Total Fat 7 g;
Saturated Fat 1 g; Sodium 135 mg

BLACK BEAN AND BUTTERNUT SQUASH CHILI   *Serves 5*

2 cups chopped onions

3 cloves garlic, chopped

2 1/2 cups chopped (1/2 inch pieces) butternut squash

4 1/2 cups cooked black beans or 3 (15 ounce) cans low sodium or no-salt-added black beans, drained

2 tablespoons chili powder

2 teaspoons ground cumin

2 1/2 cups low sodium or no-salt-added vegetable broth

1 1/2 cups diced tomatoes

1 bunch Swiss chard, tough stems removed, chopped

Add all ingredients except Swiss chard to a large pot. Bring to a boil, reduce heat and simmer, uncovered, until squash is tender, about 20 minutes.

Stir in Swiss chard; simmer under chard is tender, about 4 minutes longer.

Per Serving
Calories 379; Protein 24g; Carbohydrates 68g; Total Fat 4.3g;
Saturated Fat 1.1g; Sodium 178mg

GOLDEN AUSTRIAN CAULIFLOWER CREAM SOUP

Serves 4

1 head cauliflower, cut into florets

3 carrots, coarsely chopped

1 cup coarsely chopped celery

2 leeks, coarsely chopped

2 tablespoons Dr. Fuhrman's VegiZest (or other no salt seasoning blend such as Mrs. Dash, adjusted to taste)

2 cups carrot juice

4 cups water

2 cloves garlic, minced

1/2 teaspoon nutmeg

1 cup raw cashews or 1/2 cup raw cashew butter

5 cups chopped kale leaves or baby spinach

Place all the ingredients except the cashews and kale in a pot. Cover and simmer for 15 minutes or until the vegetables are just tender. Steam the kale until tender. If you are using spinach there is no need to steam it; it will wilt in the hot soup.

In a food processor or high-powered blender, blend two-thirds of the soup liquid and vegetables with the cashews until smooth and creamy. Return to the pot and stir in the steamed kale (or raw spinach).

Per Serving
Calories 351; Protein 12 g; Carbohydrate 45 g; Total Fat 17 g;
Saturated Fat 3 g; Sodium 164 mg

SALAD DRESSINGS AND DIPS

RUSSIAN FIG DRESSING   *Serves 2*

3 tablespoons black fig or balsamic vinegar

1/3 cup pasta sauce, low sodium or no-salt-added

3 tablespoons raw almond butter or 1/3 cup raw almonds

2 tablespoons raw sunflower seeds

Blend all ingredients in a food processor or high-powered blender until smooth.

Per Serving:
Calories 118; Protein 3 g; Carbohydrate 13 g; Total Fat 7 g;
Saturated Fat 0.8 g; Sodium 4 mg

CAESAR SALAD DRESSING   *Serves 4*

6 cloves garlic, roasted

2/3 cup unsweetened soy, almond or hemp milk

1/3 cup raw cashew butter or 2/3 cup raw cashews

1 1/2 tablespoons nutritional yeast

1 tablespoon plus 1 teaspoon fresh lemon juice

2 teaspoons Dijon mustard

black pepper, to taste

Preheat the oven to 350 degrees. Break the garlic cloves apart, leaving on the papery skins. Roast for about 25 minutes or until soft.

When cool, remove the skins and blend with the remaining ingredients in a food processor or high-powered blender until creamy and smooth.

May be used for a veggie dip or pour over 2 chopped heads (12 cups) of romaine for a Caesar Salad for two.

Per Serving:
Calories 154; Protein 6 g; Carbohydrate 9 g; Total Fat 11 g;
Saturated Fat 2 g; Sodium 86 mg

ALMOND BALSAMIC VINAIGRETTE   *Serves 6*

6 cloves garlic, unpeeled
1/2 cup water
1/3 cup balsamic vinegar
1/4 cup raw almonds or 1/8 cup raw almond butter
1/4 cup raisins
1 teaspoon dried oregano
1/2 teaspoon dried basil
1/2 teaspoon onion powder

Preheat oven to 350 degrees. Roast unpeeled garlic in a small baking dish for about 25 minutes or until soft.

When cool, remove skins and blend with remaining ingredients in a food processor or high-powered blender.

Per Serving:
Calories 77; Protein 2g; Carbohydrates 10g; Total Fat 3.1g;
Saturated Fat 0.2g; Sodium 6mg

ORANGE SESAME DRESSING/DIP   *Serves 4*

3 oranges, peeled and quartered

2 tablespoons unhulled sesame seeds

1/4 cup raw cashews or 1/8 cup raw cashew butter

3 tablespoons Dr. Fuhrman's Blood Orange Vinegar
or balsamic vinegar

Blend all ingredients in a high-powered blender until
smooth and creamy.

Add some orange juice to thin, if necessary.

Per Serving:
Calories 127; Protein 3 g; Carbohydrate 15 g; Total Fat 7 g;
Saturated Fat 1 g; Sodium 3 g

BLUEBERRY POMEGRANATE DRESSING   *Serves 4*

2 cups fresh or frozen and thawed blueberries

1/2 cup pomegranate Juice

1/4 cup raw cashews

1/4 cup raw sunflower seeds

4 tablespoons Dr. Fuhrman's Blueberry Vinegar or
other fruity vinegar

Blend all ingredients in a high-powered blender until
smooth and creamy.

Per Serving:
Calories 162; Protein 4 g; Carbohydrate 19 g; Total Fat 9 g;
Saturated Fat 1 g; Sodium 5 g

TASTY HUMMUS   *Serves 4*

1 cup cooked garbanzo beans or canned,
no-salt-added or low sodium

1/4 cup water

1/4 cup raw unhulled sesame seeds

1 tablespoon lemon juice

1 tablespoon Dr. Fuhrman's VegiZest
or other no salt seasoning, adjusted to taste

1 teaspoon Bragg Liquid Aminos
or low sodium soy sauce

1 teaspoon horseradish

1 small clove garlic, chopped

Blend all ingredients in a high-powered blender until creamy smooth.

Serve with raw and lightly steamed vegetables or as a filling ingredient with a whole grain wrap or pita.

Per Serving:
Calories 127; Protein 6 g; Carbohydrate 15 g; Total Fat 6 g;
Saturated Fat 0.7 g; Sodium 79 mg

ISLAND BLACK BEAN DIP   *Serves 4*

  1 1/2 cups cooked black beans or 1 (15 ounce) can
  no-salt-added or low sodium

  2 teaspoons no-salt-added salsa

  1/4 cup scallions, minced

  1 1/2 tablespoons Dr. Fuhrman's Blood Orange or
  other fruity vinegar

  2 tablespoons Dr. Fuhrman's MatoZest or other
  no salt seasoning, adjusted to taste

  2 tablespoons minced red onion

  1/2 cup finely diced mango

  1/4 cup diced red bell pepper

  1 tablespoon fresh, minced cilantro,
  for garnish

Remove 1/4 cup of the black beans and set aside. Place
remaining beans in a blender or food processor. Add
salsa, scallions, vinegar and MatoZest. Puree until
relatively smooth. Adjust seasonings to taste. Transfer
to a bowl and add the reserved black beans, red onion,
mango and red bell pepper. Mix well and chill for 1 hour.
Garnish with cilantro. Serve with raw vegetables.

Per Serving:
Calories 106; Protein 6 g; Carbohydrate 21 g; Total Fat 0 g;
Saturated Fat 0 g; Sodium 39 mg

SALADS

DIJON VINAIGRETTE ASPARAGUS   *Serves 4*

2 pounds asparagus, tough ends removed
1/2 cup water
1/4 cup balsamic vinegar
1/4 cup walnuts
1/2 cup raisins
1 teaspoon Dijon mustard
2 cloves garlic, pressed
2 tablespoons chopped red onion
2 tablespoons pine nuts, lightly toasted*

Place asparagus in a large skillet; add 1/2 inch of water. Bring to a boil, reduce heat; cover and simmer for 3-5 minutes until crisp-tender.

Drain asparagus and arrange in a shallow dish. Combine water, vinegar, walnuts, raisins, mustard and garlic in a food processor or high-powered blender, stir in red onion and pour over asparagus. Let stand at room temperature for 1-2 hours before serving.

Sprinkle with pine nuts before serving.

* Note: Lightly toast pine nuts in a 300 degree oven for 3 minutes, or until lightly toasted.

Per Serving:
Calories 104; Protein 7 g; Carbohydrate 14 g; Total Fat 3 g;
Saturated Fat 0.3 g; Sodium 108 mg

KALE SALAD WITH AVOCADO AND APPLES   *Serves 4*

1 bunch kale, tough stems and center ribs removed

1 avocado, peeled and chopped

2 tablespoons lemon juice

3 cloves garlic, minced

1 teaspoon fresh ginger root, minced

1/2 medium onion, minced

1 large apple, cored and chopped

Roll up each kale leaf and slice thinly. Add to bowl along with avocado and lemon juice. Using your hands, message lemon juice and avocado into kale leaves until kale starts to soften and wilt and each leaf is coated, about 2 to 3 minutes.

Mix in garlic, ginger, onion and apple.

Per Serving:
Calories 319; Protein 12g; Carbohydrates 39g; Total Fat 17.1g;
Saturated Fat 3.3g; Sodium 92mg

BUTTERNUT SQUASH SALAD
WITH TOASTED PUMPKIN SEEDS
Serves 2

4 cups butternut squash, peeled and cubed

1/2 teaspoon black pepper, divided

2 medium shallots, minced

2 tablespoons balsamic vinegar

1 teaspoon Dijon mustard

10 cups (about 10 ounces) mixed baby greens

3 tablespoons raw pumpkin seeds, lightly toasted*

Preheat oven to 350 degrees.

Arrange squash in a single layer on a jelly roll pan lightly coated with cooking spray or olive oil. Sprinkle with 1/4 teaspoon black pepper.

Bake for 35 minutes or until squash is tender and lightly browned, stirring every fifteen minutes. Remove from heat, keep warm.

Water saute shallots until tender. In a small bowl, whisk together shallots, remaining 1/4 teaspoon pepper, balsamic vinegar and Dijon mustard.

Place salad greens in a large bowl. Drizzle vinegar mixture over greens; toss gently to coat. Arrange on serving plates, top with warm butternut squash and pumpkin seeds.

* *Toast pumpkin seeds in a 300 degree oven for 4 minutes, or until lightly toasted.*

Per Serving:
Calories 239; Protein 8g; Carbohydrates 43g; Total Fat 6.6g;
Saturated Fat 1.3g; Sodium 101mg

MAIN DISHES

CREOLE CHICKEN
WITH BROCCOLI AND SPINACH   *Serves 4*

8 ounces boneless naturally raised hormone-free
chicken breasts, sliced thinly crosswise

1 cup chopped celery

1 1/2 cups chopped fresh tomatoes or canned diced
tomatoes, low sodium or no-salt-added

10 ounces frozen broccoli, thawed

1 cup chili sauce, low sodium or no-salt-added

1/2 cup chopped onion

1 large green pepper, chopped

2 cloves garlic, minced

1 tablespoon chopped fresh basil or 1 teaspoon dried

1 tablespoon chopped fresh parsley or
1 teaspoon dried

1/8 - 1/4 teaspoon dried crushed red pepper

4-5 cups fresh baby spinach

2 cups cooked brown and/or wild rice

Spray deep nonstick skillet with cooking spray or wipe
with a small amount of olive oil and heat. Cook thin
strips of chicken on medium high, turning occasionally,
for 3-5 minutes until no longer pink.

Add remaining ingredients except spinach and rice, bring to a boil and reduce heat to medium. Simmer covered for 15 minutes or until vegetables are tender. Add spinach and continue cooking until wilted.

Serve over brown and/or wild rice.

Per Serving:
Calories 359; Protein 23 g; Carbohydrate 65 g; Total Fat 3 g;
Saturated Fat 0.6 g; Sodium 148 mg

SPICY THAI BRAISED KALE AND TOFU   *Serves 4*

16 ounces firm tofu, drained well,
cut into 1 inch cubes

1 cup finely chopped onion

1 tablespoon grated fresh ginger

1 small jalapeno pepper, seeded and minced

1 teaspoon chili powder

2 cups no-salt-added or low-sodium vegetable broth

1/2 cup unsalted natural peanut butter

2 tablespoons tomato paste

2 tablespoons Dr. Fuhrman's MatoZest (or other no salt seasoning blend, adjusted to taste)

1 bunch kale, tough stems and center ribs removed and leaves chopped

1 tablespoon fresh lime juice

4 scallions, thinly sliced

Preheat the oven to 350° F.

Place tofu cubes on a lightly oiled baking dish and bake for 30 minutes, turning after 15 minutes.

Heat a large sauté pan and add onion, ginger, and jalapeno pepper. Cook until onion has softened, adding 1-2 teaspoons of water as needed to prevent sticking. Add chili powder and cook one more minute.

Whisk in vegetable broth, peanut butter, tomato paste, MatoZest and bring to a boil. Gradually add kale a few handfuls at a time, stirring to let it wilt down. Add baked tofu, cover, reduce heat, and simmer for 15 minutes or until kale is tender. Stir in lime juice and top with sliced scallions.

Per Serving:
Calories 397; Protein 18g; Carbohydrates 41g; Total Fat 19g;
Saturated Fat 2.9g; Sodium 158mg

Pasta with Roasted Vegetables, Tomatoes and Basil   *Serves 6*

2 red bell peppers, cut into 1/2 inch pieces

1 medium eggplant, unpeeled,
cut into 1/2 inch pieces

1 large yellow crookneck squash,
cut into 1/2 inch pieces

1 1/2 cups peeled butternut squash,
cut into 1/2 inch pieces

2 tablespoons olive oil, divided

1 pound whole wheat penne pasta

2 medium tomatoes, cored, seeded, diced

1/2 cup chopped fresh basil or 1 1/2 tablespoons dried

2 tablespoons balsamic vinegar or 1 tablespoon fresh
lemon juice

2 cloves garlic, minced

Preheat oven to 400 degrees. Spray large roasting pan
with nonstick cooking spray or wipe with a small amount
of olive oil. Combine red bell peppers, eggplant, yellow
squash, and butternut squash in prepared pan. Drizzle
with 1 tablespoon olive oil and toss to coat. Roast until
vegetables are tender and lightly browned, stirring
occasionally, about 25 minutes.

Meanwhile, cook pasta and drain, reserving 1/2 cup
cooking liquid.

Combine pasta, roasted vegetables, tomatoes and basil in large bowl. Add remaining tablespoon of oil, vinegar and garlic. Toss to combine. Add cooking liquid by tablespoons to moisten, if desired.

Per Serving:
Calories 365; Protein 14 g; Carbohydrate 71 g; Total Fat 6 g;
Saturated Fat 1 g; Sodium 14 mg

No Pasta Zucchini Lasagna   *Serves 8*

FOR THE TOFU RICOTTA:

16 ounces firm tofu, drained well

1/4 cup nutritional yeast

2 teaspoons lemon juice

2 tablespoons minced shallots

1 clove garlic, minced

1/2 cup fresh basil, chopped

2 tablespoons Dr. Fuhrman's MatoZest (or other no salt seasoning blend, adjusted to taste)

1 teaspoon dried oregano

2 teaspoons ground chia seeds

dash black pepper

FOR THE VEGETABLES:

2 heads broccoli, coarsely chopped

4 cups sliced mixed fresh mushrooms (such as shiitake, cremini, oyster)

4 medium bell peppers (red, yellow and/or orange) seeded and chopped

7 ounces baby spinach

FOR THE LASAGNA:

4 cups no-salt-added or low sodium pasta sauce, divided

2-3 medium zucchini, sliced lengthwise into thin slices

shredded fresh basil for garnish

Preheat oven to 350 degrees.

To make the tofu "ricotta", place the tofu in a bowl and mash until crumbly. Add remaining ingredients and mix until well-combined and the consistency resembles ricotta cheese. Set aside.

To prepare the vegetables, saute the broccoli, mushrooms, bell peppers and spinach without water, over low heat for 5 minutes or just until tender.

To assemble the lasagna, spread a thin layer of the pasta sauce on the bottom of a baking dish. Layer the zucchini slices, sauteed vegetables and tofu "ricotta" and then spread with pasta sauce. Repeat the layers, ending with the tofu "ricotta". Spread the remaining pasta sauce on top and bake uncovered, for approximately 45 minutes, or until hot and bubbly. Garnish with the shredded basil.

Per Serving:
Calories 240; Protein 12g; Carbohydrates 39g; Total Fat 6.7g;
Saturated Fat 0.9g; Sodium 106mg

BEAN ENCHILADAS   *Serves 6*

1 medium green bell pepper, chopped and seeded

1/2 cup sliced onion

8 ounces no-salt-added tomato sauce, divided

2 cups cooked pinto or black beans or
canned no-salt-added or low sodium

1 cup frozen corn, thawed

1 tablespoon chili powder

1 teaspoon ground cumin

1 teaspoon onion powder

1 tablespoon chopped cilantro

1/8 teaspoon cayenne pepper, or to taste

6 corn tortillas

Saute green pepper and onion in 2 tablespoons of the
tomato sauce, until tender. Stir in the remaining tomato
sauce, beans, corn, chili powder, cumin, onion powder,
cilantro, and cayenne (if using). Simmer for 5 minutes.
Spoon about 1/4 cup of the bean mixture on each tortilla
and roll up. Serve as is or bake for 15 minutes in a 375
degree oven.

Per Serving:
Calories 185; Protein 9 g; Carbohydrate 37 g; Total Fat 2 g;
Saturated Fat 0.3 g; Sodium 32 mg

CALIFORNIA CREAMED KALE   *Serves 4*

2 bunches kale, leaves removed from tough stems and chopped

1 cup raw cashews or 1/2 cup raw cashew butter

1 cup unsweetened soy, hemp or almond milk

4 tablespoons onion flakes

1 tablespoon Dr. Fuhrman's VegiZest, or other no-salt seasoning adjusted to taste

Place kale in a large steamer pot. Steam 10-20 minutes until soft.

Meanwhile, place remaining ingredients in a high-powered blender and blend until smooth.

Place kale in colander and press to remove excess water. In a bowl, coarsely chop and mix kale with the cream sauce.

Note: Sauce may be used with broccoli, spinach, or other steamed vegetables.

Per Serving:
Calories 269; Protein 12 g; Carbohydrate 25 g; Total Fat 16 g;
Saturated Fat 3 g; Sodium 78 mg

LEMON ZEST SPINACH   *Serves 4*

1 1/4 pounds fresh organic spinach

6 cloves garlic, minced

5 tablespoons pine nuts lightly toasted*

3 teaspoons lemon juice

1 teaspoon olive oil

1/2 teaspoon lemon zest

Steam spinach and garlic until spinach is just wilted.

Place in bowl and toss in remaining ingredients.

Toast pine nuts in a 300 degree oven for three minutes, or until lightly toasted.

Per Serving:
Calories 123; Protein 6 g; Carbohydrate 8 g; Total Fat 9 g;
Saturated Fat 1 g; Sodium 113 mg

DESSERTS

CREAMY BANANA WALNUT ICE CREAM — *Serves 2*

2 ripe bananas, frozen*
1/3 cup vanilla soy, hemp or almond milk
2 tablespoons walnuts

Blend all ingredients together in high-powered blender until smooth and creamy.

Note: Freeze ripe bananas at least 24 hours in advance. To freeze bananas, peel, cut in thirds and wrap tightly in plastic wrap.

Per Serving:
Calories 172; Protein 4 g; Carbohydrate 30 g; Total Fat 6 g; Saturated Fat 1 g; Sodium 23 mg

BERRY COBBLER — *Serves 2*

1 banana, sliced
1 cup frozen mixed berries
dash cinnamon
few drops vanilla extract

Put banana into a small microwave safe bowl. Add frozen berries on top. Sprinkle with cinnamon and add vanilla. Microwave for about 2 minutes. Serve warm.

Per Serving:
Calories 79; Protein 1 g; Carbohydrate 20 g; Total Fat 0 g; Saturated Fat 0 g; Sodium 2 mg

WILD APPLE CRUNCH   *Serves 8*

6 apples, peeled and sliced
3/4 cup chopped walnuts
8 dates, chopped
1 cup currants or raisins
3/4 cup water
1/2 teaspoon cinnamon
1/4 teaspoon nutmeg
juice of 1 orange

Preheat oven to 375 degrees.

Combine all ingredients except the orange juice. Place in a baking pan and drizzle the orange juice on top.

Cover and bake for about one hour until all ingredients are soft, stirring occasionally.

Note: You can also simmer this in a covered pot for 30 minutes on top of the stove, stirring occasionally.

Per Serving:
Calories 207; Protein 5 g; Carbohydrate 37 g; Total Fat 7 g;
Saturated Fat 0.7 g; Sodium 4 mg

AVOCADO CHOCOLATE PUDDING *Serves 4*

1 ripe avocado, peeled, pit removed

1/2 to 3/4 cups water (start with a 1/2 cup and add more if needed to blend)

4 tablespoons natural non-alkalized cocoa powder

7 medjool dates

dash vanilla extract

Blend all ingredients in a Vita Mix or other high-powered blender.

Per Serving:
Calories 199; Protein 3g; Carbohydrates 38g; Total Fat 7.3g;
Saturated Fat 1.3g; Sodium 5mg

REFERENCES

1. Keehan, S. et al. "Health spending projections through 2017, The baby boomer generation is coming to Medicare. Health Aff. 2008 Mar; 27(2):w145-w155.

2. Gardner CD, Coulston A, Chatterjee L, et al. The effect of a plant based diet on plasma lipids in hypercholesterolemic adults: a randomized trial. Ann Intern Med. 2005;142 (9):725-733. Tucker KL, Hallfrisch J, Qiao N, et al. The combination of high fruit and vegetable and low saturated fat intakes is more protective against mortality in aging men than is either alone: The Baltimore Longitudinal Study of Aging. J Nutr. 2005; 135 (3):556-561.

3. U.S. Centers for Disease Control and Prevention. http://www.cdc.gov/nchs/data/hus/hus11.pdf#100

4. U.S. Centers for Disease Control and Prevention. http://www.cdc.gov/nchs/data/hus/hus11.pdf#99

5. Roger VL, Fo AS, Lloyd-Jones DM, et al. American Heart Association Statistics Committee and Stroke Statistics Subcommittee. Heart disease and stroke statistics-2012 update: a report from the American Heart Association. Circulation. 2012 Jan 3; 125(1):e2-e220.

6. Fulgoni VL 3rd, Keast DR, Bailey RL, Dwyer J. Foods, fortificants, and supplements: Where do Americans get their nutrients: J Nutr. 2011 Oct; 141(10):1847-54.

7. Fuhrman J, Sarter B, Glaser D, Acocella S. Changing Perceptions of Hunger on a High Nutrient Density Diet. Nutrition Journal 2010; 9:51.

8. Svendsen M, Blomhoff R, Holme I, Tonstad S. The Effect of an increased intake of vegetables and fruit on weight loss, blood pressure and antioxidant defense in subjects with sleep related breathing disorders. Euro J Clin Nutr. 2007; 61:1301-1311. Ello-Martin JA, Roe LS, Ledikwe JH, et al. Dietary energy density in the treatment of obesity: a year-long trial comparing two weight loss diets. Am J Clin Nutr. 2007: 85(6):1465-1477. Howard BV, Manson JE, Stefanick ML, et al. Low-fat dietary pattern and weight change over seven years: The Women's Health Initiative Dietary Modification Trial. JAMA. 2006; 295(1):39-49

9. Halberg O, Johansson O. Cancer trends during the 20th century. J Aust Coll Nutr Environ Med 2002; 21(1):3-8.

10. Liu RH. Potential Synergy of phytochemicals in cancer prevention: mechanism of action. J Nutr. 2004; 134(12) Suppl):3479S-3485S. Weiss JF, Landauer MR. Protection against ionizing radiation by antioxidant nutrients and phytochemicals. Toxicology 2003; 189(1-2):1-20. Carratu B, Sanzini E. Biologically-active phytochemicals in vegetable food. Ann 1st Super Sanita. 2005; 41(1):7-16

11. Hu FB. Plant-based foods and prevention of cardiovascular disease: an overview. Am J Clin Nutr. 2003 Sep;78 (3 suppl):544S-551S. Campbell TC, Parpia B, Chen J.

Diet, lifestyle, and the etiology of coronary artery disease: The Cornell China Study. Am J Cardiol 1998 Nov 26; 82(10B):18T-21T. Fujimoto N, Matsubasyashi K, Miyahara T, et al. The risk factors for ischemic heart disease in Tibetan highlanders. Jpn Heart J. 1989 Jan; 30(1):27-34. Tatsukawa M, Sawayama Y, Maeda N, et al. Carotid artherosclerosis and cardiovascular risk factors: A comparison of residents of a rural area of Okinawa with residents of a typical suburban area of Fukuoka, Japan. Atherosclerosis 2004; 172(2):337-343.

12. Hu FB, Willett WC. Optimal diets for prevention of coronary heart disease. JAMA. 2002 Nov 27; 288(20):2569-2578. Esselstyn CB. Resolving the coronary artery disease epidemic through plant-based nutrition. 2001 Autumn; 4(4): 171-177.

13. Lawton CL, Burley VJ, Wales JK, Blundell JE. Dietary fat and appetite control in obese subjects: weak effects on satiation and satiety. Int J Obes Metab Disord. 1991; 17(7): 409-416. Blundell JE, Halford JC. Regulation of nutrient supply: The brain and appetite control. Proc Nutr Soc. 1994; 53(2): 407-418. Stamler J, Dolecek TA. Relation of food and nutrient intakes to body mass on the multiple risk factor intervention trial. Am J Clin Nutr. 1997; 65(1 Suppl): 366s-373s.

14. Fontana L, Partridge L, Longo VD. Extending healthy lifespan-from yeast to humans. Science. 2010 Apr 16; 328(5976):321-6.

15. Mattes RD, Donnelly D. Relative contributions of dietary sodium source. J Am Coll Nutr. 1991 Aug; 10(4): 383-93.

16. US Department of Health & Human Services, US Food & Drug Administration, Mercury Levels in Commercial Fish and Shellfish, http:/www.fda.gov/Food/FoodSafety/Product-SpecificInformation/Seafood/FoodbornePath/ogensContaminants/Methylmercury/ucm115644.htm.

NOTES

FOR MORE INFORMATION, VISIT:

www.DrFuhrman.com

Dr. Fuhrman's official website for information,
recipes, supportive services, and products

OR CALL:

800-474-WELL (9355)